BRITAIN'S HERITAGE

Nurses and Nursing

Dr Susan Cohen

AMBERLEY

First published 2019

Amberley Publishing
The Hill, Stroud
Gloucestershire, GL5 4EP

www.amberley-books.com

ISBN 978 1 4456 8328 7 (paperback)
ISBN 978 1 4456 8329 4 (ebook)

British Library Cataloguing in Publication Data.
A catalogue record for this book is available from
the British Library.

Typesetting by Aura Technology and Software
Services, India. Printed in the UK.

Contents

1
Introduction

Nursing has been called the oldest of arts and the youngest of professions, and caring for the sick certainly has powerful historical, cultural and traditional roots.

Did you know?

The Latin word *nutrire* means to nourish, and the noun 'nurse' developed from this. By the sixteenth century it came to mean, amongst other things, 'a person, but usually a woman who waits upon or tends to the sick'. During the nineteenth century it had grown to include 'training of those who tend to the sick' and 'carrying out of such duties under the direction of a physician'.

From ancient Greece, when family members provided care, through the Holy Roman Empire and the Dark Ages, when healers practiced their art, to the tending of the sick by members of secular and religious orders, women have been at the forefront of caregiving.

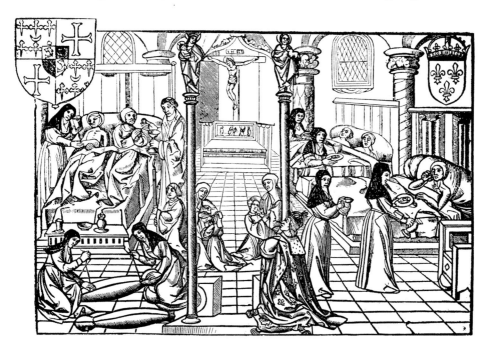

The Hotel Dieu, a medieval hospital ward with religious nursing orders. (Wellcome Library, London)

Caring for the sick came to be seen as a Christian vocation, and in Catholic countries nuns were the main providers. Whilst their nursing skills developed, progress was much slower amongst Protestants and the care of sick people in their communities was largely neglected. By the mid-nineteenth century industrialisation had driven masses of poor people from rural areas into overcrowded cities seeking work, separating them from their communities. The outcome was that many folk found themselves living in abject poverty in appalling conditions, victims to every prevailing illness, especially the deadly waterborne cholera. Most had no access to any form of medical attention or care, and

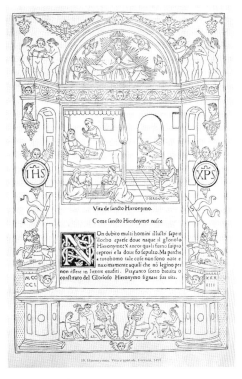

Right: Medieval nursing, from *Vita e epistole*, 1497. (Wellcome Library, London)
Below: A midnight scene at the Reichenberg Railway Station, Bohemia, where Sisters of St Vincent de Paul are tending to the wounded soldiers, c. nineteenth century. (Wellcome Library, London)

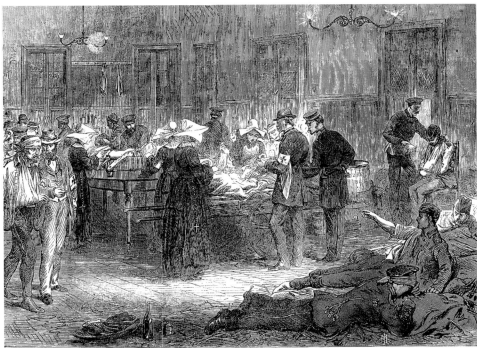

THE WAR : A MIDNIGHT SCENE AT THE REICHENBERG RAILWAY STATION, BOHEMIA.—SKETCHED BY OUR SPECIAL ARTIST.—SEE NEXT PAGE.

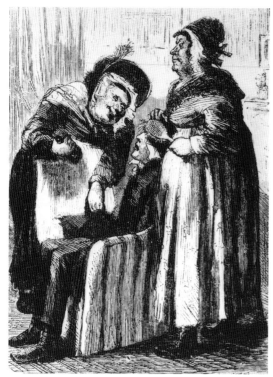

SAIREY GAMP AND BETSEY PRIG PREPARE THEIR PATIENT FOR A JOURNEY.

Sairy Gamp illustration for Charles Dickens's *Martin Chuzzlewit*. His early Victorian monthly nurse and midwife was a 'handywoman' the 'female functionary, a nurse, a watcher' who was more often than not drunk, and would request her clients 'to leave the bottle on the chimley-piece and let me put my lips to it when I am dispoged'. (Wellcome Library, London)

with no friends or neighbours to help them, they had to rely on charity or the Poor Law. Even where a parish employed a so-called nurse, she had no qualifications, her duties were unclear and had little to do with administering medical care. Nurse Philpot in Bath was one such person, and her activities included dispensing senna and salts, for which she was allowed money to buy brimstone and treacle. The alternative were services provided by charitable organisations, especially those with a religious connection, such as the Society of Protestant Sisters of Charity and the Quakers. But regardless of who was providing care, the picture was one of incompetence and ignorance. Nursing care was, at its best, basic, administered by women whose status, like that of Charles Dickens's 1844 character Sairey (Sarah) Gamp, was no better than a domestic servant.

It was thanks to a number of socially minded and philanthropic people in Britain and Europe (who recognised the need for reform) that by the mid-1800s improvements began to be made. In Germany a number of deaconess training schools for nurses were established, the best known of which was the Deaconess Institute at Kaiserwerth, Germany, set up by Pastor Fliedner and his wife Friederike in 1836. Their three-year course trained women to provide nursing and healthcare, albeit very basic, to the poor in their own homes, and was to have an impact on many future nurse reformers in Great Britain. An early visitor, in 1838, was the Quaker philanthropist and prison reformer Elizabeth Fry (1780–1845), who two years later established the Institution of Nursing Sisters in London.

She was followed, in 1850, by Florence Nightingale (1820–1910), who came away from Kaiserwerth convinced that suitably motivated women of any class could be trained as nurses and that training did not have to be organised, like Fry's, on the lines of 'sisterhoods'.

Elizabeth Fry's work had already influenced the future of nursing as a suitable occupation for educated women, with new sisterhoods appearing around the country. The Sisterhood of the Holy Cross was set up in London's St Pancras in 1845 and, in 1856, united with the Devonport Society of the Sisters of Mercy, est. 1848, creating the Society of the Most Holy Trinity, but the religious zeal of the enterprise caused many problems. By then Professor Robert Bentley Todd

SA 10N

INSTITUTION OF NURSING SISTERS,

4. DEVONSHIRE SQUARE, BISHOPSGATE, N.E.

Under the Patronage of

HER LATE MAJESTY THE QUEEN DOWAGER,

HER ROYAL HIGHNESS THE DUCHESS OF GLOUCESTER,

AND

HER GRACE THE DUCHESS OF SUTHERLAND.

DATE, *14 Jan 9* 186 *4*

This day the Sister *Palmer*

has been sent on the recommendation of

to nurse in the case of *Mrs Jones*

Signed *J. Sweet* *Lady Superintendent.*

The Committee consider £1. 1s. per week to be a suitable charge for the attendance of the Sisters, but trust by the further liberality of the wealthy, they may be enabled to grant their important assistance to those whose means are limited, also to the poor, which is the benevolent object of this Institution. Applications must be made to the Committee for all cases of Consideration, previous to engaging a Nurse.

IT IS PARTICULARLY REQUESTED :

1st.—That the Nursing Sisters should in no case be informed of the sum paid to the Institution for their services, and that no fees be given them : as from motives of delicacy, it is desirable they should not know when their services bring nothing to the Institution, or what amount of remuneration is made.

2nd.—From the same motives it is particularly requested that no present, except a book of small value, be offered to any Sister, each having entered into a solemn engagement with the Committee to refuse it, lest they should be tempted to feel discontent when any such reward to themselves is withheld. But a Superannuated Fund is open for general subscriptions and donations for the benefit of Sisters who are past work.

3rd.—Sisters accepting Legacies from Patients, are ineligible for this fund.

4th.—Travelling expenses and washing defrayed by the family employing the Sister. In infectious cases, parties are requested to pay the Sister 15s. for lodging, as, for the safety of the Home, Sisters cannot be allowed to return to it until danger of infection has ceased.

5th.—If the Services of the Sister be required beyond the period of six weeks, it is requested that at the end of that time, a communication be made, either by letter or personally, and the remuneration forwarded to the Superintendent, at the Home, 4, Devonshire Square.

Superintendent's report, June 1849. Elizabeth Fry's Institution of Nursing Sisters started out in 1840 as the Society of Protestant Sisters of Charity. Her enterprise provided young women from the lower social classes with three months of training at Guy's and various other London hospitals. (Wellcome Library, London)

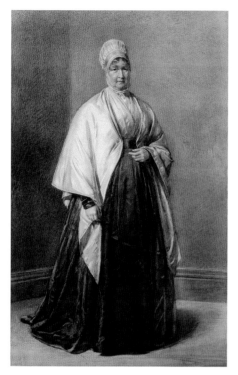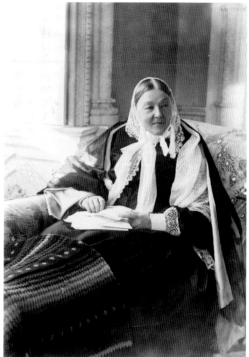

Above left: Elizabeth Fry. Colour photogravure after G. Richmond, 1843. (Wellcome Library, London)
Above right: Florence Nightingale. William Rathbone relied heavily upon her opinion, and wrote of how he submitted all his plans to her 'as we went along', *c*.1895. (Wellcome Library, London)

had set up St John's House training institution for nurses at King's College Hospital, London, and this school was proving very successful, not least of all because religious influence was studiously avoided, making the school more acceptable to wider society. From the outset, in 1848, trainees lived and learnt at the school, and the appointment of Mary Jones (1813–87) as 'Lady Superintendent' in 1853 was inspirational, as she undertook to train and dispatch parties of sisters and nurses to serve under her great friend, Florence Nightingale. Some of Miss Fry's nurses were also amongst those whom Miss Nightingale took with her to Scutari.

Did you know?

Florence Nightingale, known as 'The Lady with the Lamp,' was one of the thirty-eight volunteer nurses who travelled to Turkey. She was reported in *The Times* as being a "'ministering angel' without any exaggeration in these hospitals, and as her slender form glides quietly along each corridor, every poor fellow's face softens with gratitude at the sight of her. When all the medical officers have retired for the night and silence and darkness have settled down upon those miles of prostrate sick, she may be observed alone, with a little lamp in her hand, making her solitary rounds".

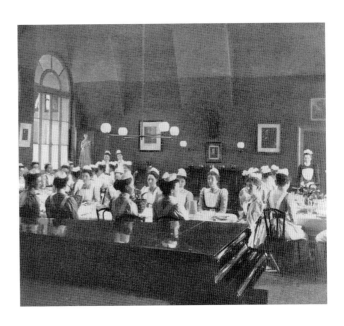

The Nightingale Home and Training School for Nurses opened its doors to trainees in July 1860, as part of the newly built St Thomas's Hospital in London. One of the first institutions to teach nursing and midwifery as a formal profession, the training school was dedicated to communicating the philosophy and practice of its founder and patron, Florence Nightingale. (Wellcome Library, London)

The public gratitude for Florence Nightingale's work running an army field hospital during the Crimean War led to the inauguration, in November 1855, of the Nightingale Fund. By 1859 there was £45,000 in the pot, and at Florence Nightingale's insistence the money was used to set up a nurses' training school at St Thomas's Hospital, London, where the matron, Mrs Wardroper, had already initiated a programme of reform. In her new role as lady superintendent, she was largely responsible for the success of the pioneering school in the early years.

Twenty years later, in July 1880, nursing reformer Eva Luckes (1854–1919) was appointed matron of the London Hospital, and her work was to have a lasting impact on nurse training. She not only addressed the inadequate numbers and quality of the nursing staff, but also developed a new training system, replacing the three years of uninstructed, unsupervised ward work with two years of practical and theoretical training including time spent on the wards. Florence Nightingale's dream of professionally trained nurses was now a reality, and was to have an impression far beyond hospital doors.

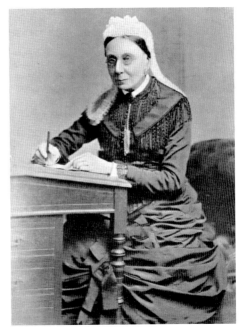

Mrs Wardroper was matron of St Thomas's Hospital from 1854 to 1887, and first lady superintendent of the Nightingale Home and Training School for Nurses between 1860 and 1887. (Wellcome Library, London)

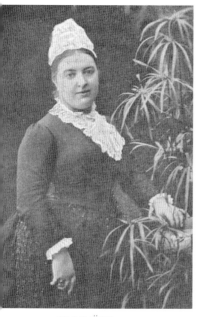

EVA C. E. LÜCKES.

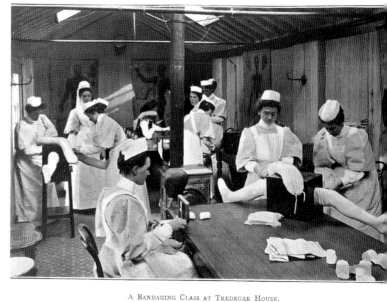

A BANDAGING CLASS AT TREDEGAR HOUSE.

The Preliminary Nurse Training School of the London Hospital.

Above left: Miss Luckes, matron of the London Hospital, which was described as 'the great hospital of the east of London'. (Wellcome Library, London)

Above right: A bandaging class at Tredegar House c.1905, the preliminary training school of the London Hospital, which was opened in 1895. (Peter Maleczek)

Below: The nurses' sitting room, Wolverhampton, c.1912. (Peter Maleczek)

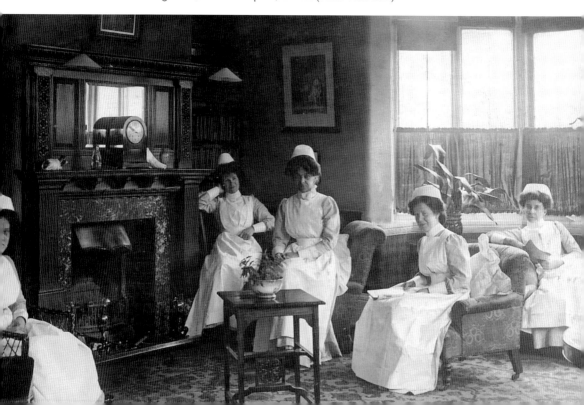

2
Community Nursing

The Birth of District Nursing

In Liverpool in 1859, Miss Robinson, a hospital-trained nurse, was engaged by William Rathbone VI (1819–1902) to care for his wife in her final days. Impressed by the benefits of professional nursing, William, a prominent local philanthropist, wondered 'what illness must mean in the homes of the poor' and to his horror discovered they lacked any healthcare. He promptly re-engaged Miss Robinson for a three-month trial to visit the sick poor in their homes and teach 'the rules of health and comfort'. The experiment almost failed but ultimately gave William the impetus to extend the service and employ more nurses. Unable to find 'women with the necessary experience and good character to be entrusted with the work' he consulted Miss Nightingale, whom he considered 'in matters of nursing, to be my Pope'. Her advice was simple, he should train them himself. Through their combined efforts – his philanthropy and her expertise – a new training school and home for nurses opened alongside the Liverpool Royal Infirmary in 1863.

With William Rathbone's concept of a hospital-trained district nurse now established, eighteen 'districts' were created across the city, and a system of local nursing associations

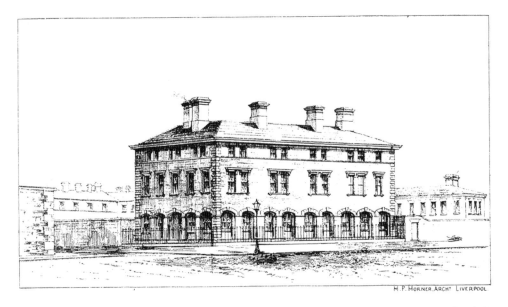

M.P. HORNER, ARCH⸀ LIVERPOOL

Liverpool Nurse Training School and Home, 1865. Miss Merryweather was appointed as the first lady superintendent, having trained at King's College Hospital and the pre-Nightingale Fund St Thomas's Hospital. (Wellcome Library, London)

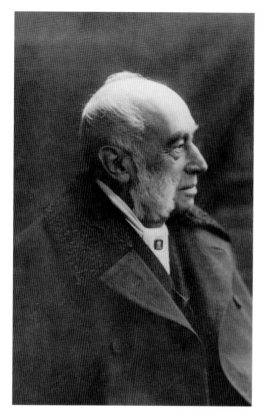

established. The Liverpool model was soon adopted elsewhere and before long district nurses were at work in other industrial towns and others, including Manchester (1864), Derby (1865) and Leicester (1867). The situation was different in London where there were a number of schemes providing care. Mrs Ranyard's Biblewomen nurses worked in the Seven Dials district but their mix of poor training, proselytising and patching-up patients was quite unsatisfactory. The East London Nursing Society was no better as it only had seven nurses and barely touched the surface

Left: William Rathbone VI, who inaugurated the idea of employing trained nurses to attend the sick poor in their own homes, was a Liberal MP and a social and welfare reformer. (Wellcome Library, London)
Below: A street group of women and children on District 3, Liverpool, c.1905. These were exactly the people who William Rathbone wanted to benefit from the new district nursing service.

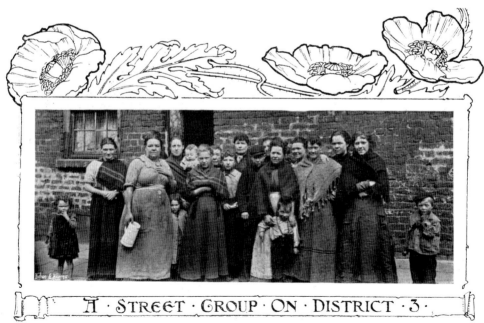

A · STREET · GROUP · ON · DISTRICT · 3 ·

of need. William Rathbone stepped in again, commissioning Miss Florence Lees (1840–1922) to carry out a survey of district nursing in London in 1874. The outcome was the establishment of the Metropolitan and National Association for Providing Trained Nurses for the Sick Poor (MNA) in Bloomsbury, with its own central home and training school, setting the standard for district nurse training in the capital.

The new enterprise needed money and funding came, unexpectedly, from Queen Victoria when she celebrated her Golden Jubilee in 1887. A sum of £70,000 was set aside from monies donated to the Women's Offering, and the newly created Queen Victoria Jubilee Institute for Nurses was inaugurated by royal charter in 1889. From the outset, any woman who wanted to undertake the six-month training course to qualify as a so-called Queen's Nurse (QN) had to have a minimum of one year's nurse training in a recognised school attached to a general hospital – this was raised to three years by 1928. District training was broad ranging and included subjects that were rarely encountered in the hospital setting. Queen's

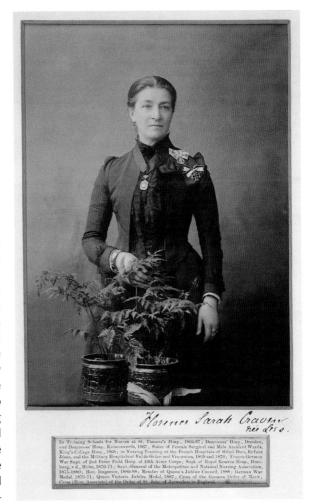

Florence Sarah Craven née Lees.

In Training Schools for Nurses at St. Thomas's Hosp., 1866-67; Deaconess' Hosp., Dresden, and Deaconess' Hosp., Kaiserswerth, 1867; Sister of Female Surgical and Male Accident Wards, King's College Hosp., 1868; in Nursing Training at the French Hospitals of Hôtel Dieu, Enfant Jésus, and the Military Hospitals of Val de Grâce and Vincennes, 1869 and 1870; Franco-German War Supt. of 2nd Fever Field Hosp. of 10th Army Corps; Supt. of Royal Reserve Hosp., Homburg, v.d., Höhe, 1870-71; Supt.-General of the Metropolitan and National Nursing Association, 1875-1880; Hon. Inspector, 1880-88; Member of Queen's Jubilee Council, 1888; German War Medal, 1870-71; Queen Victoria Jubilee Medal, 1887; Cross of the German Order of Merit; Cross (Hon. Associate) of the Order of St. John of Jerusalem in England.

Florence Lees was a highly trained nurse herself, and insisted that district nurses had a higher level of training than ordinary nurses, and that they should be accountable to a superintendent. (Wellcome Library, London)

Nurses learnt about sanitation, plumbing, infection control and the importance of fresh air as well as subjects ranging from cooking for convalescents to making blinds to shade windows. Above all, they needed to be adaptable and innovative – essential requirements for caring for folk often in the most adverse conditions.

The scene was now set for the new QNs to care for the sick poor in their own homes, and Florence Lees's handbook, *Guide to District Nurses and Home Nursing*, proved to be invaluable in the national development of district nursing.

Meanwhile, William's influence had helped establish St Patrick's Home for District Nurses in Dublin in 1876, whilst in Scotland Mrs Higginbotham set up the Glasgow Sick and Poor Private Nursing Association in 1875.

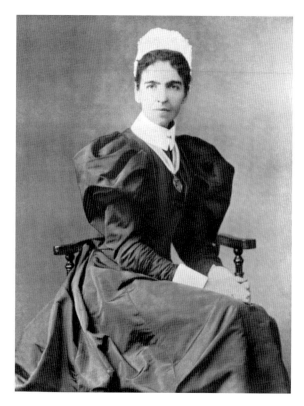

Dame Rosalind Paget (1855–1948) was William Rathbone's niece and a trained nurse. She was the first Queen's Nurse and inspector, 1890–91. (Wellcome Library, London)

Rural District Nursing

The poorest folk in rural areas across the country had even less nursing care than their city counterparts, but their plight improved thanks to another pioneering reformer, Mrs Elizabeth Malleson (1828–1916), who set up an experiment in home nursing in the isolated hamlet of Gotherington, Gloucestershire, in 1883. She raised money herself to pay for a nurse to be trained, then established the first rural nursing association. The QVJIN Rural District branch was constituted in 1888, and new county nursing associations were soon set up across the country. Life was not easy for the rural district nurse for she lived an isolated life, often in lodgings under the watchful and critical eye of a landlady. There were 'Books of Association' to maintain, which included a casebook, a large register of cases and a time book, and like her town counterpart, she was subject to regular inspection by a superintendent. Her work load could be huge, as Nurse Milford found out in 1910. The five parishes she covered in her Gloucestershire district had a population of just 1,400, but this was spread across an area of around 12 square miles, and many of the roads were treacherous. In her first year she paid 3,243 visits to 127 medical cases and eighty-six surgical cases, and had twenty-seven nights on duty. It all proved to be too much for her and after two years she reluctantly resigned. The rural district nurses' patients were very varied, and included hop pickers, travellers in caravans and crofters in the remotest parts of Scotland, many of whom were difficult to reach. Very many of the earliest nurses used a donkey and cart, which had to be abandoned in very bad weather. They wrote of tramping across muddy fields and of battling against snow blizzards to reach a patient, so it is no wonder that the application form for prospective rural

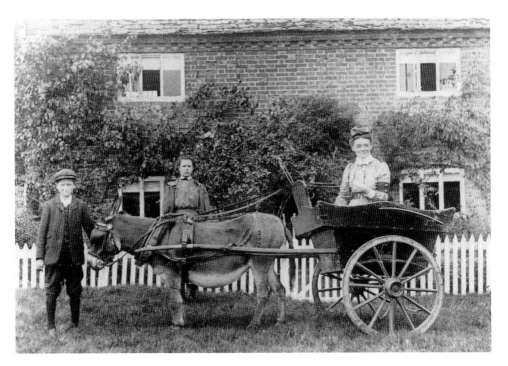

Above: District Nurse Jenny Wolfe in her donkey cart in Gotherington, Gloucestershire, c.1890. (QNI)

Below left: The Lady Dudley district nurse is seen here visiting a poor patient in Bealadangan Connemara, Ireland, c.1910. The hovel has no chimney or windows and the only place for the smoke from the fire to escape is via the entrance. (QNI)

Below right: Health visitor visiting a poor household, c.1900. (Wellcome Library, London)

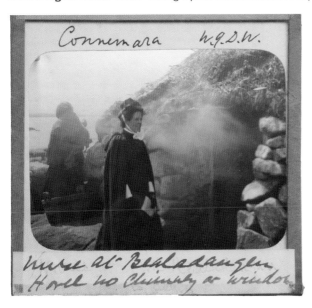

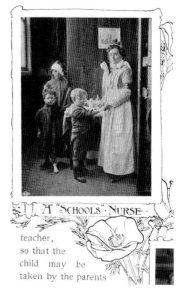

nurses asked, 'Are you a good walker and accustomed to the country?' Before the provision of cars, these rural nurses relied on every imaginable form of transport from ponies and horses, bicycles and motorcycles to rowing boats.

The district nurse was accustomed to poverty and insanitary living conditions, especially in rural Ireland. When one nurse attended a maternity case in 1910 she found 'a house in an old stable. There is no bed ... just a table, one chair and one stool ... Patient is lying in one corner in a frightful condition'. But the hardest thing the nurses had to deal with was 'superstition combined with old customs as regards the sick'. One district nurse wrote of how her patient abandoned the prescribed treatment for an ulcerated leg after a few days in favour of a 'large piece of moss, with earth attached to it, lace on the open sore, with the earthen side next to it'. It was no wonder the wound did not heal.

Public Health Nursing: Health Visiting and School Nursing

Did you know?

Few people know that Florence Nightingale was also responsible for the first programme of education for health visitors, and for promoting its spread. Indeed, in 1892 she wrote of the importance of health visiting in rural, as well as urban, areas, pointing out the sad fact that 'there are more people to pick us up when we fall, than to enable us to stand upon our feet'.

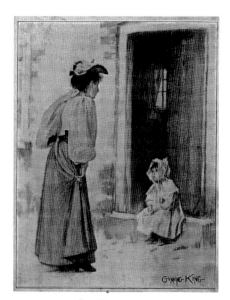

EARLY RESPONSIBILITIES.

DISTRICT VISITOR—" Tell your mother I want to see her, dear."
SMALL CHILD—" She's out."
DISTRICT VISITOR—" Well, then, go and call one of your sisters."
SMALL CHILD—" Please, they're all gone out."
DISTRICT VISITOR—" What, and left you at home alone ? "
SMALL CHILD—" I'se got to mind the baby."

When the Manchester and Salford Ladies Health Society set up a local home visiting service in 1862, they were motivated by the idea of spreading health knowledge among women and children. Little did they realise that they were laying the foundation for a future health visiting service in Britain. In 1916 the Royal Sanitary Institute began overseeing qualifying courses for health visitors, and when nurse registration was introduced in 1919, the newly created Ministry of Health established the first statutory health visiting qualification.

Community nurses soon found themselves working in schools. The Metropolitan and National Nursing Association sent their first QN into the Vere Street Board School in 1891, and before long 'a nurse visited the school

A school nurse in Liverpool, 1905. In 1895 Mrs William Rathbone paid for a nurse to attend the minor ailments of school children, and within nine months 1,000 children had been seen.

every morning and spent between one and two hours seeing twenty–forty children and dealing with burns, cuts, abscesses, opthalmia etc. as well as examining for dirt and vermin'. In 1904 the education committee in Widnes appointed a district nurse to 'attend to the minor ailments of children, both for their sakes as a curative measure, and also to secure a higher attendance'. A formal school medical service was introduced as a result of the 1907 Education (Administrative Provisions) Act, and once again Liverpool was in the vanguard of social progress, for in 1909 two of the nurses on ordinary district work attended a school for one day a week. As the *British Journal of Nursing* remarked in August 1908, the new Education Act 'opened up a new field to the nursing profession, and it is certain that the service will require a type of nurse adequately trained and possessing in a marked degree the characteristics of tact and keen observation'.

Poor Law Nursing

Whilst Florence Nightingale's early reforms in nursing were taking place at St Thomas's Hospital, London, the poorest in society had to rely on the workhouse infirmary. These were squalid and neglected places where pauper inmates acted as untrained 'nurses' and was a situation that William Rathbone wanted to change. In 1864 he offered money anonymously for the Liverpool workhouse to employ trained nurses in the infirmary, and in spring 1865 Miss Nightingale sent her most able St Thomas's nurse, Agnes Jones (1832–68), yet another Kaiserwerth trainee, to act as lady superintendent at the Brownlow Hill Workhouse Infirmary, along with twelve Nightingale nurses. Thanks to Agnes's pioneering work, by 1878 pauper assistants were no longer used in workhouse infirmaries. Then, in 1879, workhouse reformer Louisa Twining (1820–1912) was instrumental in setting up the Association for Promoting Trained Nursing in Workhouse Infirmaries to train and supply nurses and to secure the appointment of trained matrons.

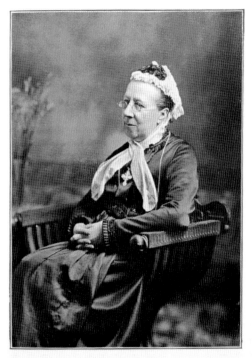

Louisa Twining (1820–1912) The association she established, under the patronage of Princess Christian, aimed to train and supply nurses and to secure the appointment of trained matrons in workhouse infirmaries. (Wellcome Library, London)

MISS LOUISA TWINING.
Pioneer of Workhouse Nursing Reform.
(*Photo: Elliott & Fry.*)

The nurse as midwife

Up until well after the introduction of the National Health Service in 1948, most women gave birth at home. Midwifery became regulated with the passing of the first Midwives Act for England and Wales in 1902, and the newly established Central Midwives Board ensured that only trained and qualified women could act as midwives. Not all nurses were midwives, but any Queen's Nurses, who were, by definition, trained nurses, and wanted to undertake maternity work – which meant most who were working in rural areas – had to pass the appropriate examination. The next major step was the establishment of nursing as a recognised profession.

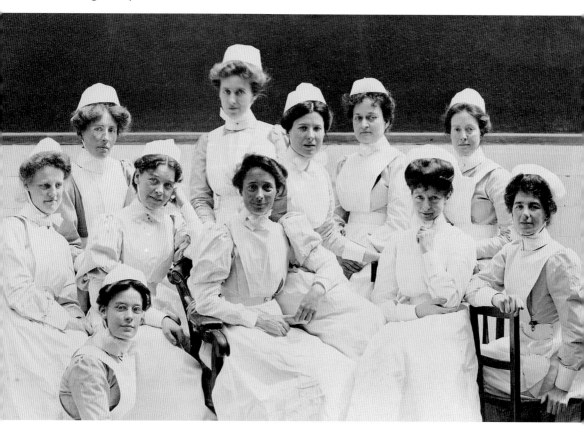

Labour ward nursing staff and pupil midwives, 1908. (Wellcome Library, London)

3
The Dawn of a New Profession

Nursing pioneers were divided on the issue of professionalising nursing. Like Florence Nightingale, Eva Luckes, matron of the London Hospital, believed that nursing was a vocation and that exams would deter many able women. But Ethel Bedford Fenwick (1857–1947), a highly experienced nurse and former matron of St Bartholomew's Hospital, held a different view and was determined to raise the status of nurses, thereby protecting the public from untrained caregivers. In her view state registration was the solution, and in 1887 she began her campaign to achieve this goal with the establishment of the British Nurses' Association, which acquired royal status in 1891. So began a lengthy battle on the one hand against doctors trying to protect their authority, and on the other hospital governors, who feared that registration would lead to organised and more expensive workers. Another crusade was started in 1915, led by Sarah Swift, matron-in-chief of the British Red Cross, who wanted a college of nursing established, with the focus on training courses and the introduction of a register of nurses. Success came soon, for the new college was founded in March 1916 and within a year the membership had grown from thirty-four to 2,553. Three years later Mrs Fenwick achieved her ambition, for on 23 December 1919 the Nurses' Registration Act was passed and three General Nursing Councils for England and Wales, Scotland and Ireland were established.

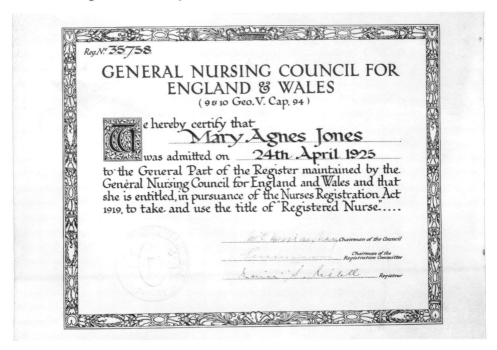

General Nursing Council Certificate, April 1925. (Science Museum, London)

For the first time in British nursing history, there was to be a register of qualified nurses, training schools would be approved and the question of pay and conditions would be dealt with on an official basis.

Well before nursing was officially professionalised, a nurse's appearance and demeanour were always considered very important, and Florence Nightingale insisted that her nurses were dressed simply and looked efficient and clean. Immediately after the Boer War, one of her students, Miss Van Rensselaer, designed a uniform that included a long blue dress, a white apron with shoulder straps and a white frilly cap that tied under the chin. Over time individual hospitals adopted their own variations, with caps, aprons, a pin, different coloured belts, piping and stripes providing information about rank and training. The nurse's cap remained a challenge to maintain for decades.

Did you know?

In the nineteenth and twentieth centuries a buckle attached to the front of her belt was the only way that a registered nurse could personalise her uniform. The designs were typically quite detailed and eye-catching, and added a beautiful touch to an otherwise somewhat plain and conservative outfit. Now they are traditionally given as a gift on graduation.

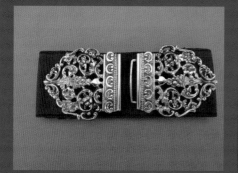

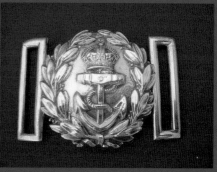

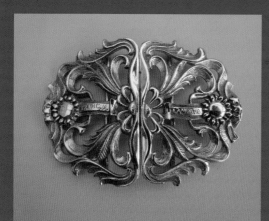

Above left: A silver nurse's buckle, hallmarked '1898'. (Peter Maleczek)
Above right: Silver buckle for a nurse with 'Queen Alexandra's Royal Naval Nursing Service, n.d'. (Peter Maleczek)
Left: A nurse's silver buckle with Royal College of Nursing motifs. The Latin motto *tradimus lampada* means 'we carry the torch'. The stars and suns symbolise the day and night service of nursing. (Peter Maleczek)

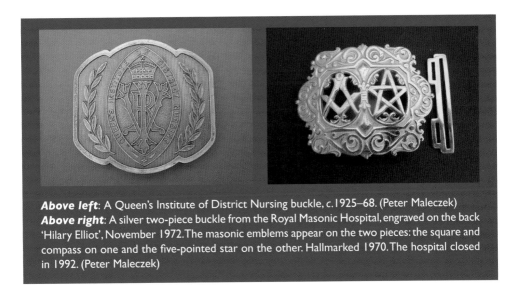

Above left: A Queen's Institute of District Nursing buckle, *c*.1925–68. (Peter Maleczek)
Above right: A silver two-piece buckle from the Royal Masonic Hospital, engraved on the back 'Hilary Elliot', November 1972. The masonic emblems appear on the two pieces: the square and compass on one and the five-pointed star on the other. Hallmarked 1970. The hospital closed in 1992. (Peter Maleczek)

Nurses at Stobhill Hospital, Glasgow, were still struggling with having to neatly pleat their starched white cotton caps, complete with drawstring, well into the 1930s. Elsewhere, nurses were subjected to headgear that had to be folded precisely or they would face the wrath of the sister, who would always notice if they were out of place. Other rules relating to appearance applied, as Zena Edmund-Jones remembered, '...hair had to be up off the shoulders and collars, nails clipped short and clean, no jewellery, no wrist watches'. Added to this, black stockings and black lace-up shoes with rubber heels were the order of the day. A key part of Marion Kirby's uniform was the heavy, woollen, black cloak with red lining, which had to be worn if she was out in public, but had the advantage, as she recalled, of keeping her 'as warm as toast in the winter'. Matrons and assistant matrons, who were renowned for ruling with an iron rod, dressed to fit their role, as trainee nurse Emily Dick recalled of the matron at Stobhill General. This lady wore 'a long-sleeved button-up frock of a bluish denim cloth, a collar of a hard starched material, topped by a starched white apron and hard white belt. When the dress sleeves were rolled up she wore frilled cotton over-sleeves with hard cotton cuffs'.

QNs had their own distinctive uniform, with strict rules applied to every aspect of their attire. In the early years they wore a brassard adorned with Queen Victoria's monogram on the left arm and a bronze or silver Queen's badge, which denoted status, hung as a pendant on a cord or ribbon. These district nurses were instantly recognisable in their floor-length dress, long outdoor cloak and familiar bonnet, but over the decades their uniform, and that of all nurses, were slowly modified to be more practical. But Miss Loane's advice, given in 1904, that every country district nurse should have 'good boots, warm light underwear, stout umbrella and the lightest possible district bag', was just as relevant in the 1950s as it was decades earlier.

There was also a strict protocol about how a nurse addressed her colleagues, and it was Mr, Mrs or Miss for consultants, and sister, staff nurse or nurse. Gossip was forbidden, and nurses were discouraged from engaging with their patients, a rule that student nurse

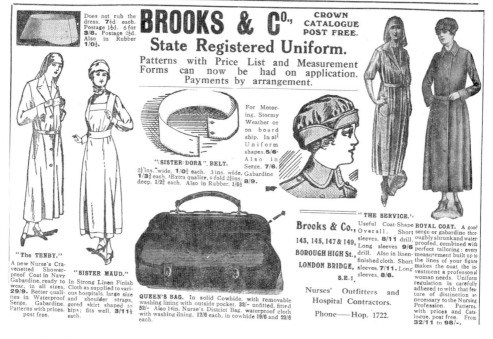
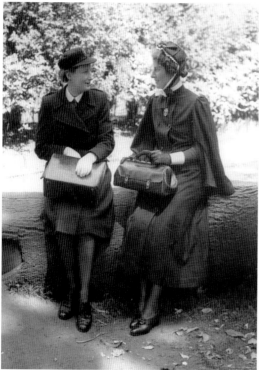

Above: Advert from *Nursing Notes*, October 1924, for SRN uniform and the district nurses' bag.
Below left: From a set of eight postcards celebrating 150 years of district nursing, and the changes in uniform. The nurse on the right (early 1900s) is wearing her badge on a cord around her neck, and leather gloves. The nurse on the left is wearing a 1950s uniform, redesigned in 1945, with the QNI badge on her cap. (Queen's Nursing Institute)

Geraldine Marchesi found very hard to abide by, especially when she was reprimanded for cuddling a crying child on her ward in the middle of the night.

From the early days, living-in was compulsory for trainee nurses. Conditions varied, and whilst some students found them very harsh, others were delighted. The nurses' home where Monica Matterson lived was a Nissen hut on the Yorkshire Moors, and was so cold with only one radiator that the water froze in the bowl by the bedside. To keep warm, the nurses would borrow long theatre socks and stone hot water bottles, but if matron did one of her customary 'raids' these were taken back, and all the nurses were in trouble. For Gladys Tubb, who was used to sharing a bed at home with one of her numerous siblings and who had only ever slept in an unheated bedroom,

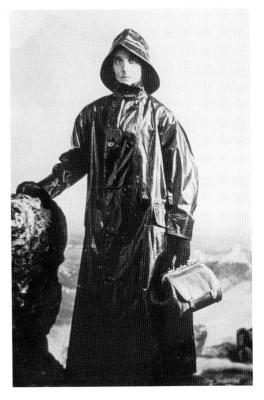

Right: A district nurse carrying her Gladstone-style 'district bag' and dressed for extreme weather in a Sou'wester. This image, taken on a glass slide, may well have been posed for in a studio, c.1910. (QNI)
Below: Several of the theatre nurses in this picture are wearing the badge of St Bartholomew's Hospital Nurses League. Other badges include the Charing Cross and Queen Mary's Hospital for the East End medals and West London Hospital Badge, c.1930s–40s. (Peter Maleczek)

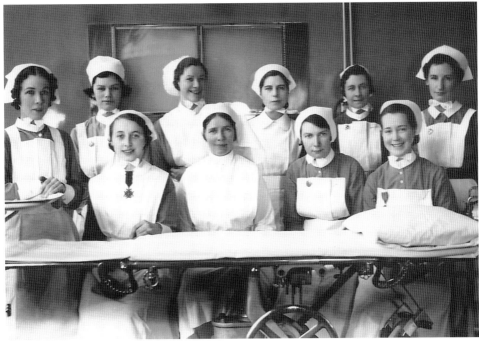

the reality of having her own room with a radiator was, as she said, 'paradise. I had privacy at last!'

As late as the 1960s the trainee nurse's life was strictly monitored, even down to being told how many pairs of socks, shoes and knickers to bring with her on arrival. Many hospitals exerted a strong Christian ethos, with daily prayers on the wards, and unless a nurse was on duty, she had to attend chapel.

Did you know?

At some hospitals, lining up beds was done with military precision. A board, or string, was laid on the floor to a line running down the length of the ward, and the beds had to be pushed exactly to the edge, with the wheels exactly pointing at each other so that no one would trip over them. Every pillow had to be in line, with the tucked in part pointing in the opposite direction to the ward entrance. Sheets were turned back to the distance between elbow and fingertip.

The practice of nurse trainees taking their meals together was deliberate, for it gave the matron the opportunity of making sure they ate properly and to dispense supplementary vitamin and iron tablets to those who she thought were not eating enough. The district nurse

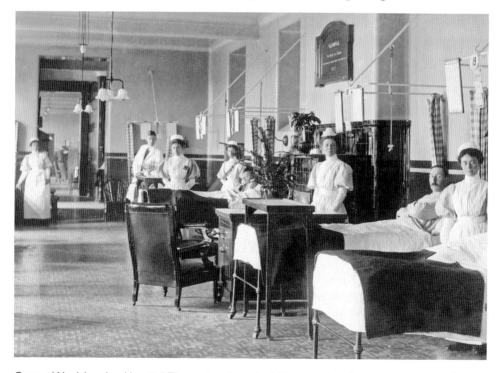

George Ward, London Hospital. The notice above bed 19 notes that the patient was on a chicken, milk and fish diet, and was under the care of Sir Bertrand Dawson. Early twentieth century. (Rob McRorie)

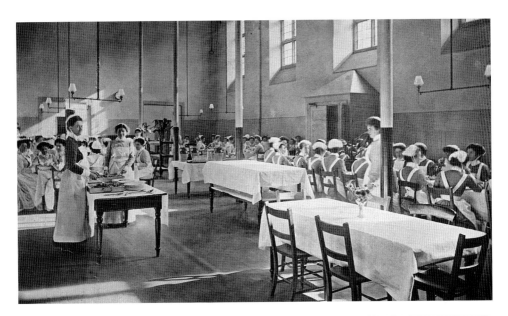

Above: The dining room at St Bartholomew's Hospital, *c.* 1908. Seated at long tables, a strict hierarchy was maintained, with matron at the top end of the sister's table and nurses arranged at long tables in descending order of seniority. (Wellcome Library)
Right: A Queen's Nurse standing by her car, a Model T Ford, *c.* 1920. (QNI)

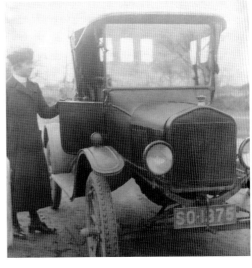

was advised by Miss Loane to have 'a good solid breakfast' and to 'never leave home for a long round without a sandwich'.

The probationer QN also lived in the nurses' home for her six months of training, under the watchful eye of the superintendent; however, once qualified and on the 'district' she was on her own, and at the mercy of what her district nursing association could afford to pay for accommodation. In rural areas, rented cottages, every bit as dilapidated as the homes of their poor patients, were not uncommon, nor were lodgings overseen by unsympathetic landladies who disliked the odd hours the nurse was forced to keep. Getting around the district to see patients was a challenge that hospital nurses did not have to contend with, and it was perfectly reasonable for the application form to ask, 'Are you a good walker and accustomed to the country?' Modes of transport changed over the decades from the pony and trap, donkey and horse to the motorcar, motorcycle and scooter. These women had to be tough, for walking miles to reach snowbound patients was par for the course in the harsh winter months. Relying on the help of a doctor was hazardous, for rough seas and bad weather could prevent him making the dangerous crossing to the remote islands off the Scottish mainland and elsewhere.

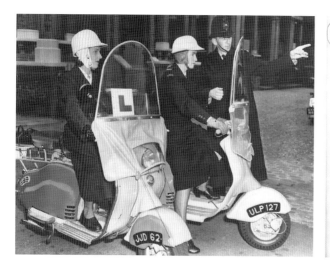

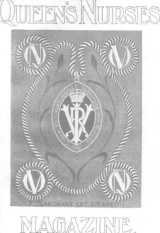

NURSING NOTES AND MIDWIVES' CHRONICLE

A PRACTICAL JOURNAL FOR MIDWIVES AND NURSES.

BEING THE JOURNAL OF

THE INCORPORATED MIDWIVES' INSTITUTE, THE ASSOCIATION OF CERTIFIED MIDWIVES,
ITS AFFILIATED ASSOCIATIONS, AND THE TRAINED NURSES' CLUB.

THE POST CERTIFICATE SCHOOL FOR MIDWIVES.
THE ASSOCIATION FOR PROMOTING THE TRAINING AND SUPPLY OF MIDWIVES.
AND THE OVERSEAS NURSING ASSOCIATION.

Office—12, BUCKINGHAM STREET, STRAND, LONDON, W.C.2

Vol. XXXVIII. No. 447	MARCH, 1925.	[Price 3d. Post free, 4d.

CONTENTS.

	PAGE		PAGE
Notes. County Council Elections. Rex v. Bateman	31	Correspondence	38
On Insobriety. Penal Session	32	Notes from Far and Near	38
The Maternity Service : Under Health Insurance Scheme	33	Central Midwives Board	39
Puerperal Sepsis	34	Practical Notes O. N.	40
Public Health Administration	35	Midwives Institute : General Meeting—Reports	41
The College of Surgeons Museum	36	Overseas Nursing Association	46
Book Notes	37		

MIDWIVES' INSTITUTE.

(Founded 1881. Incorporated 1880)

THE ASSOCIATION OF CERTIFIED MIDWIVES AND
TRAINED NURSES' CLUB,

12, Buckingham Street, W.C.2.

March, 1925.

4th, Friday, 6.30 p.m.—Executive Council and Club Committee.
13th, Friday, 4 p.m.—Executive Council and Committee of Affiliated Associations.
20th, Friday, 6 p.m.—House Committee.
" " 7 p.m.—Social Evening. Hostess : Miss I. Hill. Miss Marsters will speak on " Business Methods," followed by discussion.
27th, Friday, 6.30 p.m.—Midwives in Council, to discuss the results of the County Council Elections.

LECTURES to prepare for the Central Midwives Board Examination twice a week (Mondays and Wednesdays, at 5 p.m.).

MIDWIVES ASSOCIATIONS.

(Affiliated to the Midwives' Institute)

East Sussex.

The next meeting will be held on Monday, March 9th at 3.15 p.m. at the Wesleyan Schoolroom, Perrymount Road, Hayward's Heath, when Miss Cancellor of the N.C.C.V.D. will speak on **Venereal Disease as a Complication of & Pregnancy**.—E. M. Wyatt, Hon. Sec.

Birmingham.

March 13th, Dr. Dain, 4.45 p.m. Subject : Menopause and Cancer. —Miss Rickford, Secretary.

Blackpool and District.

The next meeting will be Wednesday, March 11th, 3 p.m.—M. Lightbown, Hon. Sec.

Bournemouth.

A meeting will be held at the G.F.S. Club, St. Peter's Road on Monday, March 2nd, at 3 p.m. Tea 6d. Speaker Miss Maude Bone, M.B., Ch.B.—I. M. C. Druitt, Hon. Sec.

Bristol.

The next meeting will be held at the Kingswood Nurses Home, Hanham Road, by kind invitation of Miss Bosworth, on March 17th, at 3.30 p.m. An address will be given by Miss Cross (Matron of The Maternity Hospital, Brunswick Square). " A Short Talk about Midwifery in Italy."—Miss Hancock, Hon. Sec.

Gosport and Fareham.

The meeting for March will be held at the " House of Industry," Gosport, 3 p.m., on the 18th. Dr. Una Mulvany of Portsmouth will Lecture. Any midwife visiting the district will be welcome.— L. M. Cryer, Hon. Sec.

ESSEX.

Southend Branch.

Wednesday, March 18th, Dr. C. A. Shields, Public Health Office, Clarence Street, 3.15 p.m.—Mrs. Tween, Secretary, 85, Stornaway Road, Southchurch.

Colchester Branch.

Tuesday, March 17th, Dr. Ryan. Ear, Nose and Throat, 71, High Street, Colchester, 3 p.m.—Miss Pearson, Secretary, Health Offices, Colchester.

Chelmsford Branch.

Saturday, March 7th, Miss Burdew, Nursing of " Chronics," 3 p.m., 125 London Road—Nurse N. Millett, Secretary.

S.E. Essex Branch.

Friday, March 13th, Miss Elsie Hall, the Midwives Opportunity, Nurses' Home, Beauchcroft Road, Leytonstone, 5.30 p.m.—Nurse Kennard, Secretary.

Saffron Walden Branch.

Tuesday, March 17th, Miss Landon, Antenatal Work, 37, West Road, 3 p.m.—Nurse Doyle and Nurse Crampton, Secretaries.

Romford Branch.

Wednesday, March 11th, Dr. Ball, Infant Feeding, Tuberculosis Dispensary, 3 p.m.—Miss Landon, Secretary, Old Cottage, Shenfield Common, Brentwood.

Hertfordshire.

A course of lectures is being given monthly by Dr. Helen Noth, at Bricket House, St. Albans, at 3.30 p.m. Next one March 19th. Tea provided after each lecture.—E. S. Cowper, Hon. Sec.

Liverpool.

March 12th : " Disorders of the Climacteric," Miss Ivens, University of Liverpool, Department of Hygiene.
March 26th : " Prevention of Ophthalmia Neonatorum," Dr. T. Stevenson, St. Paul's Eye Hospital.

Maidstone.

Tuesday, March 3rd, at 3 p.m., at Sessions House, Dr. Ponder, Assist. M.O.H., will lecture on the Infant.—H. Wells, Hon. Sec.

Portsmouth.

Next meeting at Welfare Centre, Fratton Road on Wednesday, March 4th, 3.45 p.m. Lecture by Dr. McCalden, Subject : " Twilight Sleep "—A. G. Phillips, Hon. Sec.

Whitefield and District.

March 12th, a lecture will be given by Dr. Hall at 2.45 p.m.—A. J. P. Hon. Sec.

S.W. London.

A Social will be held on Monday, March 2nd, at 7 p.m., at 47 Lavender Gardens. Members and friends are invited.—C. A. Tiflin, Hon. Sec.

Southampton and District.

A meeting will be held at the Municipal Clinic on Wednesday, March 11th, at 6 p.m. Report of Representative.—E. Harvey, Hon. Sec.

Cornwall.

The next meeting will be on Saturday, March 28th, at the Infant Welfare Centre, Lemon Quay, Truro, at 3 . p.m. Lecture by Dr. Burnell commencing 3.15 p.m.—Ethel Lyon, Hon. Sec.

North Middlesex.

Next meeting Wednesday, March 11th, at 260, Fore Street, Edmonton. Dr. Ash will give his second lecture, which unavoidably had to be postponed.—M. Andrews, Hon. Sec.

Above left: London district nurses P. Ebril of Limerick, Ireland, and C. Franklin of London, receive directions from a policeman before making their rounds on motor scooters, c.1957. The London County Council was experimenting with the use of scooters to speed the nurses on their visits to patients throughout the city. (Peter Maleczek)
Above right: Queen's Nurses' Magazine, 1909.
Left: Nursing Notes and Midwives' Chronicle, 1925.

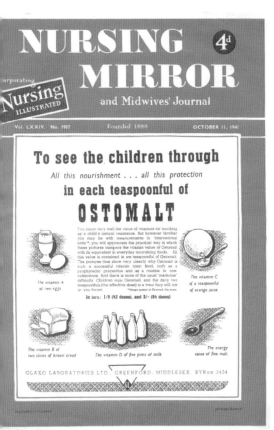

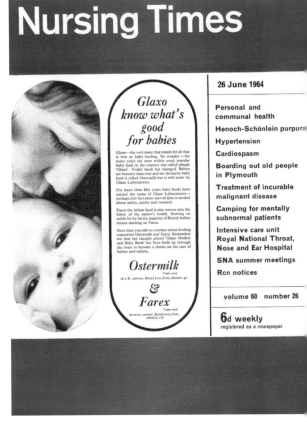

Above left: *Nursing Mirror*, 1941.
Above right: *Nursing Times*, June 1964.

Nurses were never short of reading material, enabling them to keep up to date with the latest goings-on in the nursing world. *The Nursing Record* and *Nursing Mirror* were launched in 1888 and had a potential readership of some 15,000 nurses, and from 1905 had competition from *Nursing Times*, the official College of Nursing journal. However, *Nursing Mirror* remained the best-selling journal among nurses, with a circulation of 31,000 in 1919. From 1904 QNs had their own journal, the *Queen's Nurses' Magazine*, in which 'questions affecting district nursing could be discussed, information with respect to developments in sick nursing given, and opinions exchanged on all questions affecting the profession'. Besides topical articles, all the publications were filled with advertisements, and both the *QNM* and *Midwives Chronicle and Nursing Notes* regularly included invalid and ration cookery recipes as well as past examination questions and model answers.

But it was, perhaps, during the First World War that the magazines came to play such an important role and kept hospital, private and district nurses in touch with their fellow professionals and boosted their morale.

4
The First World War

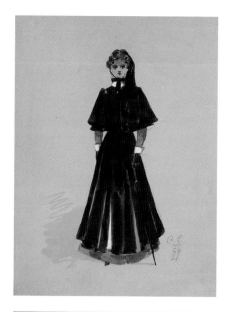

Providing nurses for wartime service was a major exercise, and the Second Boer War (1899–1902) was the first time that nurses were deployed in any numbers. Before then, some nurses worked for the Army Nursing Service (est. 1881) with their numbers boosted by reservists from Princess Christian's Army Nursing Service Reserve (PCANSR) (est. 1897).

The Boer War highlighted the inadequate supply of nurses – the PCANSR had only sixty-five serving nurses in 1902 – and as a result

Left: A watercolour image of an army hospital nurse in her outdoor uniform, c.1899. (Wellcome Library, London)
Below: Miss C. Wills and other QNs who were working for the Territorial Force Nursing Service (TFNS) at the First Eastern General Hospital, Cambridge. (QNI)

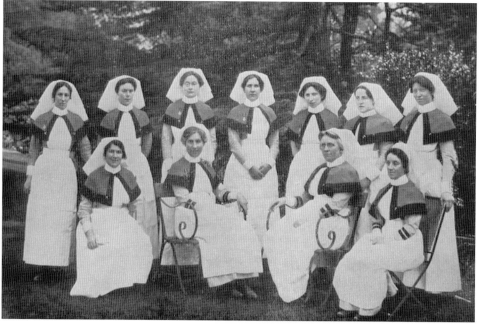

was reformed (post-war) as Queen Alexandra's Imperial Military Nursing Service (QAIMNS). A reserve corps was created in 1908, and the following year a new Territorial Nursing Force Service (TFNS) was set up at home, comprising matrons, sisters and staff nurses, all aged under forty-five. They had to sign a three-year contract and received either an annual £5 retaining fee or, if working, a scaled allowance. Nurses made an annual commitment to the War Office and carried on working in civilian posts in peacetime, but were ready to be mobilised to work in the twenty-five Territorial Force hospitals and auxiliary units if war was declared. In addition, in 1911 the newly established Civil Hospital Reserve attracted a further 600 trained nurses.

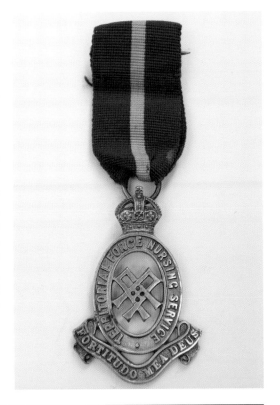

A TFNS badge bearing the motto *Fortitudo Mea Deus*, which translates as, 'The Lord is my Strength.'

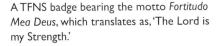

Did you know?

Famous VADs included Agatha Christie, who initially worked as a VAD nurse and then dispenser from October 1914 until September 1918 at Town Hall Hospital, Torquay; Vera Brittain, writer and peace campaigner, who joined the VADs in September 1915 and worked as a nurse in various military hospitals on the home front, on Malta and from early August 1917 until the end of April 1918 at No. 24 General Hospital, Étaples, France, until March 1919; and Naomi Mitchison (née Haldane), Scottish novelist and poet, who became an auxiliary VAD nurse at St Thomas's Hospital, London in August 1915, and resigned when she got married in 1916.

At the outbreak of war in 1914 Miss Maud McCarthy, QAIMNS and matron-in-chief for the British Army, had 516 regular and reserve nurses under her command, but by the end of the year, the numbers of reservists had attracted more than 2,200 women. The numbers were boosted by nurses from New Zealand, Canada and Australia, and by the end of 1915 had an additional 557 highly qualified QNs who were given leave of absence from the QVJIN for the duration of hostilities.

No matter how well qualified a nurse was, none were prepared for, or trained to deal with, war casualties. *Nursing Times* wasted no time in including special articles

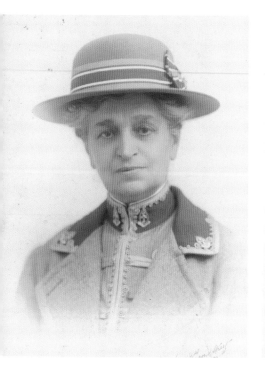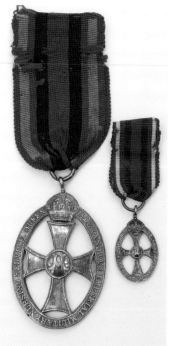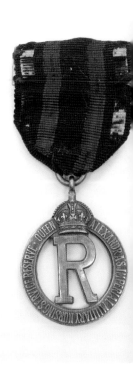

Left: Miss Maud McCarthy (1858–1949) of the Queen Alexandra Imperial Military Nursing Service. By the time the Armistice was signed in November 1918, she had about 6,400 nurses under her command. She was appointed GBE in 1918. (Museum of Military Medicine)
Middle: QAIMNS badge.
Right: QAIMNS Reserve badge.

on gunshot wounds, burns and the accompanying shock, and later on the effects of gas. Letters published in the nursing journals gave readers a flavour of the dangers the nurses faced at home and abroad. Sister Reid wrote of how, in France in late 1914, she narrowly escaped a German bomb that was dropped from an aeroplane close to her carriage on an ambulance train. The *British Journal of Nursing* recorded that several nurses had gone to do fever work with the Serbia Relief Fund and the Scottish Women's Hospital Unit in Serbia, and not surprisingly, were not immune to falling victim to illness themselves. Sadly, several, including Miss Louisa Jordan, succumbed to typhus, from which she died in early 1915. Ever resourceful, and rather than stand idle, when the fever cases in one Serbian unit began to fall off, the nurses started a baby clinic and dispensary for children, providing an invaluable service to poor mothers, many of whom had repeatedly fled from the enemy and fallen victim to hunger and fatigue. Danger was never far away, but nurses accepted this as part of their lot. Writing from a Clearing Station in France, in 1915, an anonymous nurse wrote of the 'daily visits by Taubes [German reconnaissance planes that carried bombs, which were thrown from the cockpit] ... I was on my way to the Chateau to call on the nurses. I heard a noise above me ... I had to take refuge in a house for it stopped and I knew bombs would be dropped. Three fell but no one was injured'.

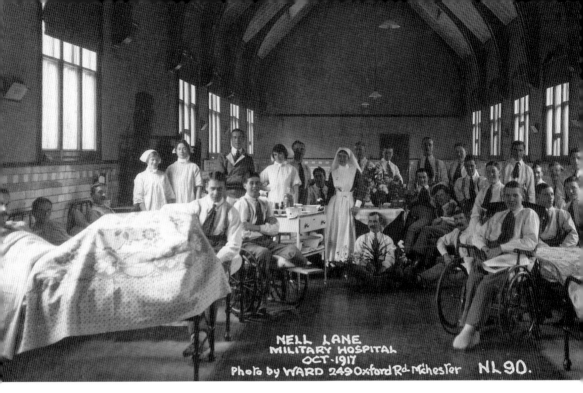

NELL LANE
MILITARY HOSPITAL
OCT·1917
Photo by WARD 249 Oxford Rd Manchester   NL 90.

Withington Hospital, Nell Lane, Manchester, became Nell Lane Military Hospital during the First World War. It was a large pavilion-style hospital, originally built in 1855 as a workhouse for the Chorlton Poor Law Union. (Rob McRorie)

Military nurses were called upon to work on hospital barges and trains, which were used to transport wounded servicemen to the coast, for evacuation to England. Nurse Tanner, a QAIMN Reservist and former London Hospital nurse and midwife, was on a barge on the Somme and captured the grim reality of injuries in her diary for 3 September 1916:

The interior of a hospital barge in which the cargo hold was converted into a functioning ward. Makeshift hand-operated lifts enabled stretchers to be lowered below, and rudimentary ventilation was provided in the roofs. Each barge had at least one QAIMNS sister, an RAMC orderly and auxiliary help, and shared an RAMC medical officer with other barges. (Wellcome Library, London)

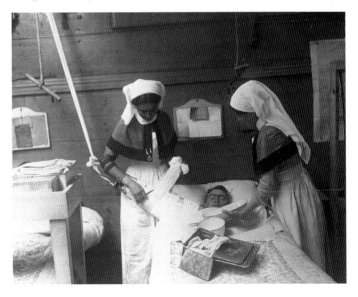

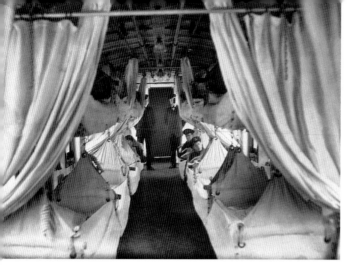

This First World War hospital train had hanging beds, which made it very difficult for the nurses to care for the patients in the upper rows. (Wellcome Library, London)

'We had several bad leg and abd [abdomen] cases, three amps [amputations] and one poor boy had both eyes shot out.' The next day she visited a hospital and saw 'one of the officers, a shell shock who could not speak or open his eyes ... they say he cannot possibly get better'.

Many of them showed great courage in the performance of their duty. Violetta Thurston and several other nurses crossed enemy lines without a permit to visit the injured in Tirlemont, Belgium, and were stopped and searched seven times before the officer realised they were English and let them pass. But Nurse Edith Cavell, who had been a superintendent of QNs in England, paid the ultimate price for helping to smuggle 200 Allied soldiers over the front line. She was captured by the German army and executed in October 1915.

Did you know?

The Florence Nightingale-designed scarlet cape, worn by the TFNS nursing sisters during the day, was intended to 'conceal the female bosom from the gaze of the licentious soldiery'. The 'T' badge identified the women as members of the TFNS.

At home, many nurses and district nurses signed up with the TFNS and the Red Cross, and were initially involved in setting up territorial and auxiliary hospitals in a range of requisitioned buildings, from stately homes and schools to universities and workhouse infirmaries. Brighton Grammar School was converted for military use, becoming the 520-bed Second Eastern General Hospital. More than a quarter of the 100 nurses were QNs and were there ready to accept their first convoy of 300 wounded men when they arrived from Mons on September 1914. Like their counterparts abroad, they encountered wounds and diseases they had never seen before. Sister Lily Ethel Nazer nursed many Sikhs and Gurkhas at Netley Auxilliary Hospital, and described the arrival of one batch:

> Five out of the last twenty were hand and arm wounds and these walked in; the other fifteen were heavy stretcher cases, some had six or eight wounds from shrapnel and three were badly frostbitten: one has since died, another developed tetanus and several amputations have had to be done. All the wounds are horribly septic on arrival but it is surprising how quickly they clean up with regular dressing and attention.

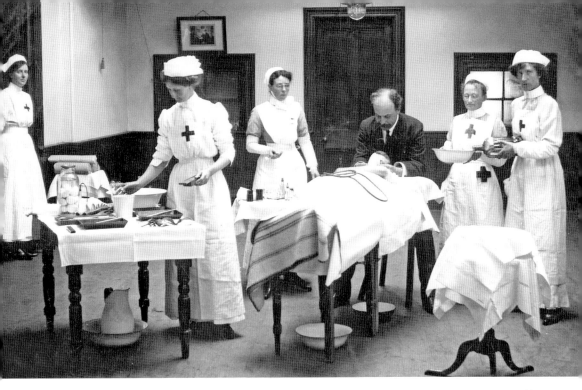

Red Cross nurses and a TFNS sister working at Sussex County Hospital, c.1915–17. (Peter Maleczek)

Nurses found themselves working in specialised units set up to treat conditions including venereal diseases, typhoid fever, consumption, dysentery and septicaemia, as well as psychological trauma, facial disfigurement and limb replacement. Possibly the most unusual place that nurses worked in during the First World War was the Endell Street Military Hospital in London, for, with the exception of some male orderlies, it was staffed entirely by women, but only treated men.

There was still a great need for nurses among the general population, and in the early years of the war every district nurse was urged to

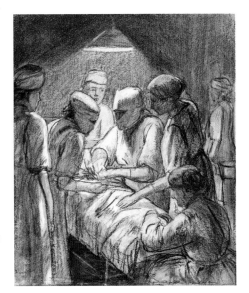

> throw herself more entirely into her sphere, to make herself indispensable to the people by identifying herself with their joys and sorrows as well as their ills, and by so doing keep awake the diminishing sympathy of those good people often a source of anxiety on the district; work so well worth doing, but unknown and unrecognized save by the discerning few.

Right: All the staff – surgeons and nurses – in this sketch are women, working at the Endell Street Military Hospital, London. Francis Dodd, 1920. (Wellcome Library, London)

Much of their work was connected with public health. In view of the possibility of bombardment, the district nursing association in Brighton assigned all their nurses to dressing and ambulance stations. St Helen's, Lancashire, had their nurses helping inoculate soldiers against typhoid, whilst across the country district nurses helped care for wounded and convalescent soldiers. Nurses were allocated to various minor injury centres in the London boroughs of Paddington and Marylebone, as well as undertaking work at the Marylebone tuberculosis dispensary. By 1916 Gloucestershire County Nursing Association reported that 'of the seventy-two District Nursing Associations affiliated to the county nursing association, sixty-four are co-operating in this scheme for Public Health Work'. A year later, there were also sixteen infant welfare centres in the county attended by the district nurses, where mothers could have their babies weighed and ask for advice on health and feeding.

In recognition of their acts of gallantry, amongst the many awards, fifty-five nurses of the QAIMNS and the TFNS received the Military Medal, but countered against this, some 200 QAIMNS members lost their lives while on active service. So many nurses were awarded the Royal Red Cross, first and second class, that one Territorial nurse commented in March 1916:

> Now that the Royal Red Cross is being showered about, amongst recent awards I note 'First Class' for the untrained and 'Second Class' for the 'paid nurse'. I used to hanker after this honour, now somehow it seems cheapened. Sour grapes, perhaps you will say.

Her complaint was indeed justified for in 1920 a new Royal Red Cross Warrant was introduced, cancelling all previous ones. The numbers to be issued were strictly restricted, for, as the *British Journal of Nursing* noted in November 1920, 'the large number given in the recent war has materially depreciated its value'.

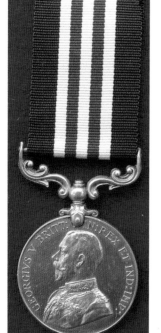

Left: The Military Medal was established by King George V in March 1916.
Below: The first class Royal Red Cross was instituted in 1883, and this silver second class Associate Royal Red Cross was added in 1915. It conferred upon women members of the nursing service, irrespective of rank.

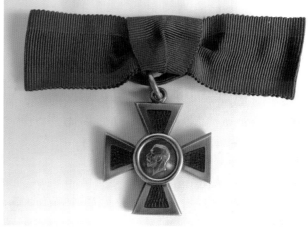

5
Between Two World Wars

The end of the First World War in November 1918 may have been a time of celebration, but for nurses the influenza pandemic that swept the country created a huge additional workload for them and put them at risk. Amongst the early casualties to succumb to the disease in 1918 were six Great Ormond Street Hospital nurses, along with five from the Edmonton Military Hospital, and the only way that nurses could be released for epidemic nursing at Gilroes Isolation Hospital, Leicester, was to temporarily close the children's ward on Anstey Lane. The Ministry of Health issued advice to nurses who were caring for victims of the illness, which included avoiding inhaling the patient's breath, keeping the patient isolated if possible, and in a warm and well-ventilated place. QNs covering Brighton, Hove and Preston treated 376 cases of influenza during 1918, and often visited patients two, three or even four times a day. In Leicester, the district nurses struggled along for the first two weeks of October 1918 without any extra help, working for between nine and eleven hours a day, and just as they thought they could not carry on any longer, help arrived.

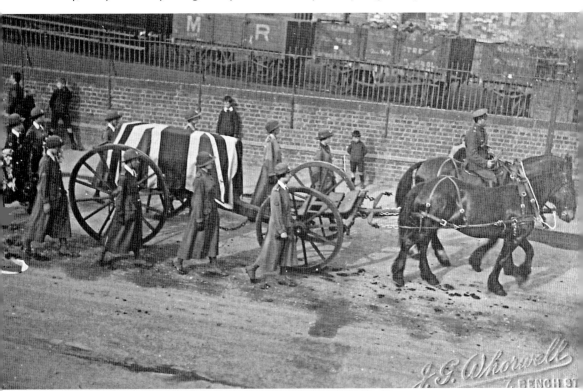

A postcard showing the funeral procession of a victim of the Spanish flu epidemic in Dover, 1918.

The 1920s marked a turning point for nursing, which was now a recognised profession. The Nurses' Registration Act 1919 set down new national nurse education standards, and once trained a nurse became a state-registered nurse. Nurse registration itself began in the UK on 30 September 1921, with five parts to the new register, covering general (female only) nurses, fever nurses, male nurses, mental nurses and sick children's nurses. Nurses had to pay an annual 'retention fee' for inclusion, set at 2s 6d in 1924, but registration remained voluntary up until the introduction of the Nurses Act in 1943.

The College of Nursing membership had increased from 2,553 in 1916 to 17,336 by 1920, and continued to grow steadily,

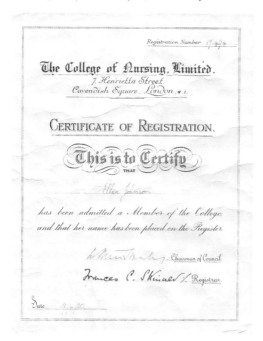

Left: Ellen Johnson's certificate of registration for the new College of Nursing, 19 April 1920. The college was granted a royal charter in June 1929, with Queen Mary as patron, but there were so many objections from other nursing organisations that they had to wait until 1939 before they could include 'Royal' in their title. (Wellcome Library, London)

Below: A page from the 1922 Register of Nurses, showing Ethel Bedford Fenwick entered as 'State Registered Nurse Number 1' in 1919. (Peter Maleczek)

REGISTER OF NURSES FOR 1922

Reg. No.	Name.	Permanent Address.	Date and Place of Registration.	Qualifications.
3944	Farr, Lucy	214, Cherryhinton Road, Cambridge	May 19, 1922, London	Cert. 1902–1905, Incorporation Infy., Southampton.
912	Farrall, Gertrude	278, Clarendon Park Road, Leicester	Nov. 18, 1921, London	Tr. 1901–1902, Sheffield Royal Hosp.
2920	Farrant, Norah	33, Chenies Street Chambers, London, W.C.1	April 21, 1922, London	Cert. 1905–1907, London Hosp.
2921	Farrell, Elizabeth Fielding	Dunsfort, Circular Road, Dungannon, Co. Tyrone, Ireland	April 21, 1922, London	Cert. 1908–1911, Sunderland Infy., Dublin.
4473	Farrer, Julia Frances	10, Colosseum Terrace, London, N.W.1	May 19, 1922, London	Cert. 1896–1899, Addenbrooke's Hosp., Cambridge.
950	Farrier, Annie Elizabeth	Brook House Farm, Wednesfield, Wolverhampton	Nov. 18, 1921, London	Cert. 1917–1920, Wolverhampton Union Infy.
4603	Farrimond, Mary	7, Wigan Road, New Springs, Wigan	June 16, 1922, London	Cert. 1907–1910, Warrington Union Infy.
433	Farthing, Margaret Ellen Eliza (née Bethell)	74, High Street, Wem, Salop	Oct. 28, 1921, London	Tr. 1900–1902, St. Olave's Union Infy., Bermondsey, London.
590	Faulkner, Ada	c/o Miss C. A. Little, 88, Spring Bank, Hull	Oct. 28, 1921, London	Cert. 1909–1912, City and County of Nottingham Workhouse Infy.
680	Faulkner, Elizabeth Jane	c/o Mrs. Arthur Middleton, Grove House, Bradford Peverell, Dorchester	Nov. 18, 1921, London	Cert. 1913–1914, Bridport Dispensary and Cottage Hosp.
679	Faulkner, Gertrude Lilian	Stamford House, Westwood, Scarborough	Nov. 18, 1921, London	Cert. 1909–1912, Salisbury Infy.
3293	Faulkner, Gwendolen Pattie	Longham Vicarage, East Dereham, Norfolk	April 21, 1922, London	Cert. 1912–1915, East Suffolk and Ipswich Hosp.
2627	Faulkner, Mary Elizabeth	34, Beechwood Avenue, Kew Gardens, Surrey	Mar. 17, 1922, London	Cert. 1899–1902, Hull Royal Infy.
5157	Faulkner, Millicent	c/o Mrs. J. H. Tracey, Elm House, Makeney, London	July 21, 1922, London	Cert. 1911–1914, District Infy., Ashton-under-Lyne.
3290	Faull, Mary Elizabeth	Douglas House, Southwold, Suffolk	April 21, 1922, London	Cert. 1903–1906, Guy's Hosp., London.
1242	Fawcett, Agnes	c/o Mrs. L. Lodge, Tuakan, Auckland, New Zealand	Feb. 3, 1922, London	Cert. 1917–1920, Southport Infy.
3945	Feacey, Ellen	17, Casewick Road, London, S.E.27	May 19, 1922, London	Cert. 1899–1902, Whitechapel Infy., London.
2922	Fearn, Lucy	130, Freedom Road, Walkley, Sheffield, Yorks	April 21, 1922, London	Cert. 1913–1917, Infy. of the City of London Union.
4804	Fearnall, Gladys	Ivy House, Filstock, Whitchurch, Salop	June 16, 1922, London	Cert. 1917–1920, Manchester Royal Infy.
2923	Fearnhead, Frances	c/o J. Fearnhead, Esq., 20, High Street, Chorley, Lancs	April 21, 1922, London	Cert. 1911–1914, Sheffield.

102

GENERAL PART

Reg. No.	Name.	Permanent Address.	Date and Place of Registration.	Qualifications.
4604	Fearnhead, Helen	c/o Miss Dunderdale, 41, Lime Street, Great Harwood, Blackburn	June 16, 1922, London	Cert. 1914–1917, District Infy., Ashton-under-Lyne.
5158	Feather, Letitia Forster	The Royal Gwent Hospital, Newport, Monmouthshire	July 21, 1922, London	Cert. 1909–1914, St. Thomas's Hosp., London.
5159	Fechtman, Emma	2, Tweed-dale Terrace, London	July 21, 1922, London	Cert. 1906–1909, Parish Royal Infy., London.
1244	Fell, Ida Elsie (née Jefferson)	c/o —. Wollen, Esq., 33, Fentham Road, Birchfields, Handsworth, Birmingham	Feb. 3, 1922, London	Cert. 1912–1916, Royal Infy., Sheffield.
3946	Fellows, Myra	Birch Heath, Chester	May 19, 1922, London	Cert. 1914–1917, Birkenhead Borough Hosp.
877	Fenner, Caroline Ellen	St. Bartholomew's, 20, Golden Lane, London, E.C.1	Nov. 18, 1921, London	Cert. 1914–1917, St. Bartholomew's Hosp., London.
3294	Fenner, Elsie Coomber	124, Watford Road, King's Norton, Birmingham	April 21, 1922, London	Cert. 1914–1917, Aberdeen Royal Infy.
3947	Fennessy, Rosetta Mary (née Watson)	c/o Mrs. E. Watson, 18, Clapton Passage, Clapton, London, E.5	May 19, 1922, London	Cert. 1912–1915, Holborn Union Infy.
1	Fenwick, Ethel Gordon (née Manson)	20, Upper Wimpole Street, London, W.1	Sept. 30, 1921, London	Tr. 1878–1879, Royal Infy., Manchester.
2050	Ferens, Margaret Sharpe	1239, Pearl Street, Alameda, California	Feb. 3, 1922, London	Cert. 1895–1900, Glasgow Royal Infy.
3528	Fergus, Minnie (née Beever)	Spring Hill, Cumberland Road, Headingley, Leeds	May 19, 1922, London	Cert. 1905–1908, Infy. of the Leeds Union.
3948	Ferguson, Fanny Helen (née Flitness)	51, Primrose Road, Birkenhead	May 19, 1922, London	Cert. 1911–1915, Derbyshire Royal Infy.
2628	Ferguson, Jenny Raeside	Lochview, Galderbank, Airdrie, Lanarkshire	Mar. 17, 1922, London	Cert. 1908–1911, Salop Infy.
117	Ferris, Joan Henrietta	26, Sussex Gardens, Hyde Park, London, W.2	Sept. 30, 1921, London	Cert. 1916–1919, West London Infy., Hammersmith.
118	Ffolliott, Hilda Rose	1, Broadwater Down, Tunbridge Wells, Kent	Sept. 30, 1921, London	Cert. 1914–1917, Metropolitan Hosp., London.
3949	Ffoulkes, Alice Elizabeth	44, St. John's Wood Terrace, Circus Road, London, N.W.8	May 19, 1922, London	Cert. 1904–1909, St. Thomas's Hosp., London.
1245	Field, Alice Ellen Monica	Lyndale, Boundary Road, Woking, Surrey	Feb. 3, 1922, London	Cert. 1907–1911, Royal Devon and Exeter Hosp., Exeter.
1246	Field, Emma Jane	103, Ashley Road, Bournemouth	Feb. 3, 1922, London	Cert. 1911–1914, King's Norton Infy., Birmingham.
681	Field, Lilian Bessie	The Infirmary, Slough, Bucks	Nov. 18, 1921, London	Cert. 1912–1914, Cheadle Union Infy., Staffs.

103

SUPPLEMENTARY PART OF THE REGISTER FOR MALE NURSES

Reg. No.	Name	Permanent Address	Date and Place of Registration	Qualifications
9	Barrett, George	63, Buckingham Gate, London, S.W.1	May 19, 1922, London	Tr. 1903–1906, Camb. Hosp., Aldershot, R.A.M.C.
16	Brown, Harry	6, Chapel Street, Scunthorpe, Lincs	Sept. 22, 1922, London	Tr. 1908–1911, R.A.M.C. Hosps.
10	Bryant, Edward Charles	72, Verdant Lane, Catford, London, S.E.6	May 19, 1922, London	Cert. 1908–1911, Royal Victoria Hosp., Netley, R.A.M.C.
13	Clark, Walter George William	c/o G. Ayton, Esq., 58, Jersey Street, Jolimont, Subiaco, near Perth, Western Australia	July 21, 1922, London	Cert. 1909–1912, Military Hosp., Coltonera, Malta, R.A.M.C.
14	Dowty, Edwin George	Hackney Union Infy., High Street, Homerton, London, E.9	July 21, 1922, London	Cert. 1918–1921, Hackney Union Infy., London.
1	Dunn, George	8, Classic Road, Derby Lane, Stoneycroft, Liverpool	Mar. 17, 1922, London	Cert. 1901–1904, R.A.M.C. Hosps.
2	Essex, George Edmund	Herrison, nr. Dorchester, Dorset	Mar. 17, 1922, London	Tr. 1914–1917, R.A.M.C. Hosps.
21	Frost, Robert Frederick Manthorp	8, Avery Hill Road, New Eltham, London, S.E.9	Oct. 27, 1922, London	Cert. 1909–1912, Royal Victoria Hosp., Netley.
23	Green, Bertie Collin	Ascot, Parkhurst, Isle of Wight	Oct. 27, 1922, London	Tr. 1914–1918, R.A.M.C. Hosps.
11	Green, William James	2 Block, 6 Quarters, H.M. Prison, Parkhurst, Isle of Wight	June 16, 1922, London	Tr. 1912–1915, R.A.M.C. Hosps.
12	Greenwood, John Sutcliffe	555, Caledonian Road, Holloway, London, N.7	June 16, 1922, London	Tr. 1901–1903, Royal Victoria Hosp., Netley, R.A.M.C.
17	Hall, Henry Harry Edwin Longhurst	21, Radbourne Road, Balham, London, S.W.12	Sept. 22, 1922, London	Tr. 1902–1905, R.A.M.C. Hosps.
18	Long, William Joseph	H.M. Prison, Ipswich	Sept. 22, 1922, London	Tr. 1918–1921, R.A.M.C. Hosps.
3	Noakes, George	20, Seafield Road, Hove, Sussex	Mar. 17, 1922, London	Tr. 1915–1918, R.A.M.C. Hosps.
4	Raggett, Herbert	24 Quarters, H.M. Prison, Durham	Mar. 17, 1922, London	Tr. 1892–1910, R.A.M.C. Hosps.
5	Rickson, Charles Walton	13, The Avenue, Brixton Hill, London, S.W.2	Mar. 17, 1922, London	Cert. 1898–1901, Station Hosp., Rawal Pindi, India, R.A.M.C.
19	Ryan, Richard Chappell	79, Gloucester Street, London, S.W.1	Sept. 22, 1922, London	Tr. 1884–1888, R.A.M.C. Hosps.

604

MALE NURSES

Reg. No.	Name	Permanent Address	Date and Place of Registration	Qualifications
20	Steele, Arthur Champion	15, The Downs Road, Belmont, Surrey	Oct. 27, 1922, London	Cert. 1919–1922, Hackney Union Infy., London.; 1914–1916.
6	Stratton, Frederick William	Hackney Union Infirmary, 230, High St., Homerton, London, E.9	Mar. 17, 1922, London	Cert. 1919–1920, Hackney Union Infy., London.
15	Stratton, Henry George	157, High Street, Homerton, London, E.9	July 21, 1922, London	Cert. 1912–1915, Hackney Union Infy., London.
7	Wadham, Charles Thomas Henry	7, Pixley Street, Burdett Road, London, E.14	Mar. 17, 1922, London	Cert. 1912–1915, Military Hosp., Tidmouth, R.A.M.C.
22	Whitcombe, Harold Octavius	5K, Quarters, Borstall Institute, Portland, Weymouth	Oct. 27, 1922, London	Cert. 1915–1919, R.A.M.C. Hosps.
8	White, Walter	16, Camp Hill, Parkhurst, Isle of Wight	Mar. 17, 1922, London	Tr. 1894–1902, R.A.M.C. Hosps.
24	Whitsed, Arthur	Male Nurses' Temperance Co-op., 8, Hinde Street, Manchester Square, London, W.1	Nov. 17, 1922, London	Tr. 1904–1907, Lucknow Military Hosp.

605

Above: The Register of Nurses 1923, Supplementary Part of the Register for Male Nurses. When the GNC opened their first Register of Nurses, men were considered a special category and very much in the minority. Practically all received their training in the military, except for Hackney Union Infirmary. (Peter Maleczek)

Right: GNC syllabus. Between 1919 and 1951 there were two alternative training courses in mental nursing. Those following the General Nursing Council route could qualify as registered mental nurses, but the Medico-Psychological Association continued to provide parallel training until 1951. (Peter Maleczek)

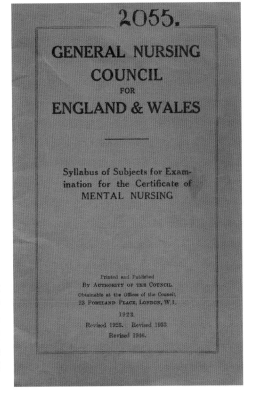

but only half of the 50,000–60,000 nurses on the state register in 1927 had joined up. Nevertheless, the college was the largest nursing organisation and had an equally impressive London headquarters, with its own club – The Nation's Nurses and Professional Women's Club – better known as The Cowdray Club. Men were eventually allowed to become associate members in 1968.

Training had moved on from the early Florence Nightingale model both in duration, which was between three and four years, and in content. In the 1920s training at the Radcliffe Infirmary, Oxford, took place at Manor House in Headington, where the probationers, as they were called, attended lectures and had practical demonstrations on dummies before they were allowed on to the hospital wards. After that, lectures had to be taken in off-duty time, which amounted to 2 ½–3 hours a day, with one whole day off every two weeks. Once qualified, an SRN could become a hospital staff nurse, an independent private nurse or work through an agency. Midwifery required a further year of training in a maternity hospital, and for QNs an additional six-month course with the QVJIN. There were also increasing opportunities for nurses to work in the public health sector as school nurses and health visitors, but it was left to local authorities to put on special courses if they wished. The College of Nursing established a public health section in 1923 and 1925 the Ministry of Health approved their six-month course for health visitors. By 1930 the college were also offering more than twenty courses covering subjects including tuberculosis nursing, venereal diseases and industrial

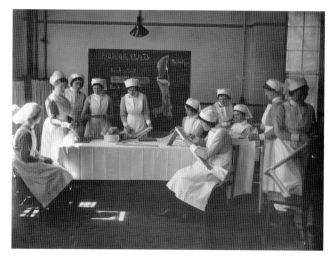

An unidentified school of nursing c.1930s. The nurses are learning how to pad splints. (Peter Maleczek)

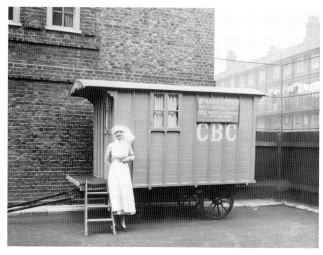

A nurse standing outside one of Dr Marie Stopes' pioneering mobile birth control clinics. The converted horse-drawn caravan travelled the country to reach as many women as possible, c.1920s. (Wellcome Library, London)

legislation, all of which had to be taken in a nurse's limited free time. Links with royalty were forged in 1926 when Queen Mary, who took a keen interest in nursing, became the official patron of the college. Three years later and, in the face of opposition from other nursing organisations, the college was awarded a royal charter, but was blocked from using the 'Royal' prefix until this was granted by King George VI in 1939.

For some, like Evelyn Prentis, who trained in the 1930s, there was a big gap between expectations and reality. Rather than being a ministering angel and soothing fevered brows, she, like almost every trainee, was set to cleaning and undertaking domestic chores, including bedpan scrubbing duty on day one, and scouring toilets the next day. Every matron knew how difficult it was to control infections and cross-infections – penicillin was only first used in 1942 – and scrupulous cleanliness was the most effective weapon at her disposal, so it was no wonder that nurses had to clean and scrub for all they were worth. Anticipation of a matron's ward round sent nurses into a spin, and even the most junior of them would be on tenterhooks. Emily Soper's superior insisted that jugs of water had to be filled to a precise level and fading flowers were not tolerated. For Josephine Chadkirk an impending inspection meant finishing tasks, or at least looking as if she had. Besides this she had to ensure that ambulant patients were seated to attention in a precise place by their bed, having been warned not to move. But there were benefits to the often dreaded ward rounds, which many nurses appreciated for they felt they offered a real opportunity to learn. Attention to detail was drummed into them, and the nurse was expected to have memorised the name, diagnosis, condition and treatment of every patient. Knowing the name of every piece of equipment was also essential: there was no trying to refer to a 'sphygmo...' when what matron wanted was 'sphygmomanometer', and the nurse had to be able to spell the word correctly.

Visiting hours offered the nurse little respite, for it freed them to get on with other important jobs. The tasks were wide ranging, from preparing individual dressings and packing them in metal containers ready for sterilising, lining up bedpans, urine bottles and sputum mugs in an orderly fashion, to sewing ward number labels into new linen, which were regularly checked by the matron. Nurses spent long hours on the ward, there were often strict controls over their private lives, and pay amounted to little more than pocket money. Added to all these privations, the fear of failing exams and the low salaries that qualified nurses received made the post of assistant nurse an attractive alternative prospect to many. The college was concerned about this, but balked against a working wage for probationers, for they were considered to be students following a professional course, who would reap the rewards when they qualified. Improvements in medical treatment and the growth in the provision of a wide range of medical services created an ever increasing demand for nurses, but there was competition as new opportunities were opening up to women, particularly in the white-collar sector, making nursing even less attractive. Every hospital experienced a high turnover of staff, not least of all because young women left on marriage. Figures produced by the Association of Nurses claimed that in 1938, of 100 entrants, thirty-eight left in the first year and only fifty completed their training. By 1930 hospitals across the country, especially the smaller ones, were struggling to attract students, precipitating two separate enquiries, the doctor-driven Lancet Commission on Nursing and the subsequent official 'Athlone' Committee in 1937. In fact the economic downturn in the early 1930s reversed the shortage of trainees, as girls were prepared to take any work they could find, even low paid nurse training.

Amongst the new recruits were a number of Jewish refugee women who managed to escape Nazi persecution in Europe, and for whom nursing was the only way to get an entry visa.

Lee Fischer, Hortense Gordon and Lisbeth Hochsinger (eventually nicknamed Hockey) had all wanted to become doctors, but were happy to settle for nurse training rather than domestic work. Lisbeth Hochsinger became a probationer at The London, and was unimpressed by how the ward sisters put her off asking questions and by the way the doctors lectured the students with 'very diluted medicine'. Whether it was an altruistic or expedient move, the Central Coordinating Committee for Refugees set up a Nursing and Midwifery Department in late 1938 to help refugee women, and over the war years and beyond between 668 and 1,000 refugees took up some form of nursing.

With war once more on the horizon, preparations were in hand to deal with casualties, and even though there were more than 80,000 nurses on the general register, there were staff shortages across the profession. The College of Nursing played a significant part in

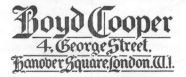
A pre-1939 advert for the College of Nursing uniform. (Peter Maleczek)

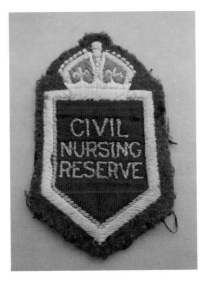
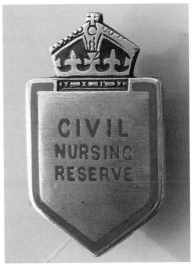

Above right and right: The woven Civil Nursing Reserve badge was worn on the left side of the uniform coat. The white metal badge was worn over the hat band.

preparations to ensure there were enough nurses available on the home front to deal with the anticipated casualties from enemy bombing. A Central Emergency Committee for the Nursing Profession was set up by the government in late 1938 to organise a Civil Nursing Reserve (CNR) and the college agreed to undertake the initial registration of nurses and auxiliaries.

Did you know?

Members of the British Red Cross and St John Ambulance Brigade were encouraged to serve in the Civil Nursing Reserve. Nursing auxiliaries could be between eighteen and fifty-five, with no previous experience, and had to be willing to take a course, which usually took the form of two weeks' theoretical and practical training in a hospital at government expense. The subjects taught were first aid, home nursing, and practical hospital work.

The CNR roll listed the volunteers, mostly retired or married nurses, who were available to be called upon in an emergency and by February 1939, 3,000 nurses had volunteered. However, enrolment was slow, possibly because of the pay structure, which meant that an auxiliary on the CNR could be earning more than her more qualified hospital counterpart.

6

The Second World War

During the Second World War nurses from every branch of the profession were called upon to contribute to the war effort, at home and abroad, but as in the previous conflict, there were insufficient trained staff to fill the demand. Unlike the previous world war there were not thousands of wounded military personnel being returned to the UK for treatment, and the casualties were largely civilians. At the outbreak there were 80,000 nurses on the general register, and Civil Nursing Reserve numbers were boosted by some 45,000 women who applied to train as nursing auxiliaries. QNs were responsible for training these women, providing instruction in basic first aid and home nursing, before their brief introduction to hospital work. CNR Irene Riley, who had previously worked in a café and cake shop, was sent to work at Richardson Military Hospital in County Durham after training and recalled that the nurses worked in shifts, including nights and 'took turns to work in the theatre, preparing and handing out the instruments'.

At home nurses were issued with gas masks, ration books and identification cards, district nurses with steel hats and respirators. Evacuation of hospitals and their patients from endangered urban areas began on 1 and 2 September 1939, and one nurse at the

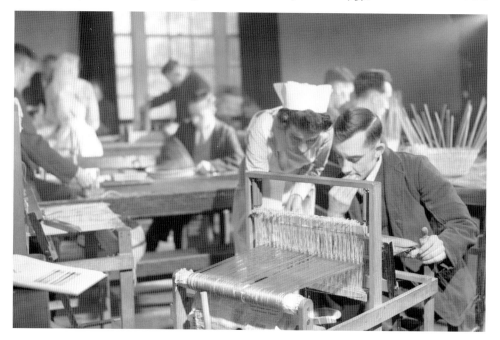

A nurse assists a convalescent soldier as he works on a piece of weaving at a loom at Mill Hill Hospital, 1942. Other soldiers can be seen in the background working on various activities, such as basket weaving. (Imperial War Museum D11979)

Student nurse Joyce Collier signs for her keys, given to her by Sister Reed at St Helier Hospital. Each student nurse had three keys – one for the door of her room, one for her wardrobe and one for her wall safe. According to the original caption, Sister Reed had been Home-Sister at the London Hospital before her retirement. She returned to nursing at the outbreak of war, due to the shortage of nurses. (Imperial War Museum D12800)

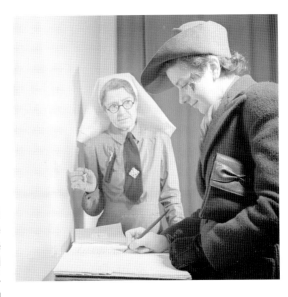

London Hospital recalled 'Red London buses and Green-Line coaches were lined up outside the Luckes Home to take patients and nurses to their temporary homes'. Inner-city hospitals had to cope with a skeleton staff, and one senior nurse remembered triumphantly how the shortage of staff afforded experienced nurses greater responsibility, writing 'on 1 March the theatres were taken over by me and are now entirely run by the nursing staff'. For newly qualified nurse Elizabeth Keogh, working at St Stephen's, Chelsea, the news that she was amongst those being loaned to another hospital came as a shock. The matron could not tell the nurses where they were going, nor for how long, only that they needed clothes for all seasons and that they might be living under canvas. Elizabeth spent the war years nursing at Horton Hospital, Epsom, working mostly on the military section. But it was all hands on deck when civilians injured during the Blitz were brought in. She remembered a very pregnant woman who got caught in an air raid whilst strolling in a local park. The baby was safely delivered. The mother had a badly broken femur, but was more worried that she had lost her glasses. Amazingly, the kindly ambulance driver went and found them stuck in a tree branch.

Wartime inevitably impacted on traditional nurse training, as student nurse Mary discovered. Instead of the usual structure, at the end of her first year she and her fellow trainees were allocated to whatever branch of nursing they showed an aptitude or interest in. For Mary, this turned

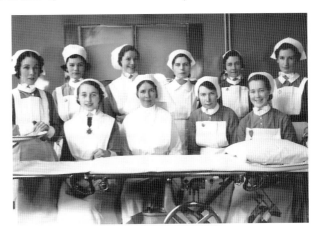

These nurses may be from one of the London hospitals, possibly St Bartholomew's, as several are wearing the badge of their Nurses League. Other nice badges include the Charing Cross and Queen Mary's Hospital for the East End medals and West London Hospital Badge, c.1930s–1940s. (Peter Maleczek)

out to be as a theatre nurse, and her experience of being on duty when a convoy of casualties arrived from North Africa in 1942 left an indelible impression:

> Most were suffering from severe and complicated leg wounds, which had been treated by casualty clearing stations at the front. The treatment comprised immobilisation of the limb in what was then called a Thomas Splint .... The discarded plaster splints and dressings were most offensive and gave off a smell which none of us working at the time will ever forget! ... We worked non-stop, as did the other theatres - from 4pm until 8am the next morning. We had the enormous satisfaction of knowing that no amputations had been necessary ... but the theatre was a sorry mess.

Did you know?

The Thomas splint was introduced in 1916 and revolutionised the way that fractures, especially of the femur, were treated. Designed by Hugh Owen Thomas, it reduced the mortality rate from 80 per cent to 20 per cent between 1916 and 1918.

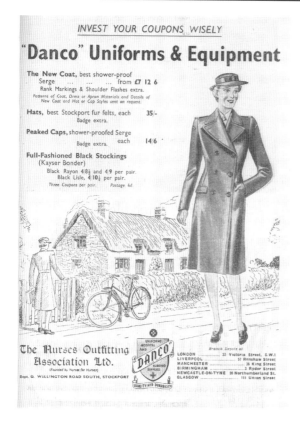

INVEST YOUR COUPONS WISELY

"Danco" Uniforms & Equipment

The **New Coat**, best shower-proof
Serge ... ... from £7 12 6
Rank Markings & Shoulder Flashes extra.
Patterns of Coat, Dress or Apron Materials and Details of New Coat and Hat or Cap Styles sent on request.

Hats, best Stockport fur felts, each   35/-
Badge extra.

Peaked Caps, shower-proofed Serge
each   14/6
Badge extra.

Full-Fashioned Black Stockings
(Kayser Bonder)
Black Rayon 4/8½ and 4/9 per pair.
Black Lisle, 4/10½ per pair.
Three Coupons per pair.   Postage 4d.

The Nurses Outfitting Association Ltd.
(Founded by Nurses for Nurses)
Dept. Q. WILLINGTON ROAD SOUTH, STOCKPORT

Branch Depots at:
LONDON .... 33 Victoria Street, S.W.1
LIVERPOOL .... 57 Renshaw Street
MANCHESTER .... 26 King Street
BIRMINGHAM .... 3 Ryder Street
NEWCASTLE-ON-TYNE 26 Northumberland St.
GLASGOW .... 111 Union Street

An advert for uniform during rationing. Clothes rationing was introduced on 1 June 1941, and ended on 15 March 1949.

During the Blitz the College of Nursing's Public Health Section set up a rota providing nursing support for the VADs and others working in Underground station shelters, and to ensure they were properly prepared, the college ran a three-day crash course. Many nurses found themselves caught up in bombing raids whilst they were on duty. Dorothy Fyles, in training at Sefton General Hospital in Liverpool in May 1941, recalled one particular night that she never forgot:

> While on duty in the Casualty Department, we heard the release of a bomb and suddenly the hospital window shattered and my nurse's cap blew off. Civilian casualties soon started to arrive – some with dreadful injuries. I remember two little boys in their pyjamas, as if asleep, but both were dead.

She never recovered her cap. From 1940, nurses were also working in

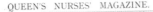

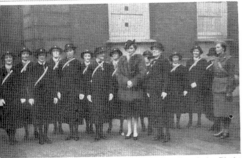

ponse that had been so evident. She also gave a brief outline of what District
rses are doing in town and country, in the bombed cities and in the reception
as.
The Duchess then inspected the various vehicles. The X-Ray unit was received
Sir Philip Chetwode on behalf of the British Red Cross Society. The Duchess
s very interested in this very valuable ambulance, which can be taken to any
ualty needing to be X-rayed, however remote may be the district where the
tric current may have failed and so rendered the hospital's X-Ray apparatus
less.
Colonel Walter Elliott, at one time Minister of Health, received the War Office
bulance, which is a splendid one with plenty of room and every convenience for
r patients.

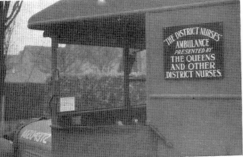

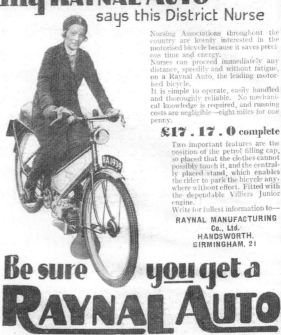

Above left: District nurses at war.
Above right: Auto-cycles and mechanised cycles like these were banned during the blackout, but to help nurses on pedal bikes be seen in the dark, in early 1940 Messrs Lunalite of London prepared a 'luminous armlet … with the word Nurse standing out in bold relief on a blue background (yellow in daylight) … The luminous effect can be re-activated by exposure to artificial light'.

factories with government contracts, and the government at last recognised that industrial nursing was a skilled branch of the profession.

District nurses made their own special contribution as part of the home-defence system, a front-line occupation. There were 4,566 QNs in 1939, and unlike in the First World War, they were discouraged from volunteering for active service. Still, many did join up and the decline in numbers was only halted by the introduction of the 1943 Control of Engagement Order, effectively preventing certain categories of nurses, including district nurses, leaving their posts. Their duties included meeting evacuated mothers, children under five and schoolchildren at railway stations, and then checking their health in case there were issues that might create a problem with their host family. Many assisted in the extra infant welfare centres and antenatal clinics that were set up. One QN wrote of how she was 'loaned' to the London County Council in October 1940 to work at a temporary

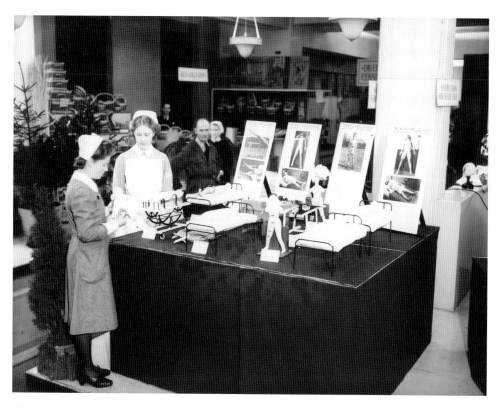

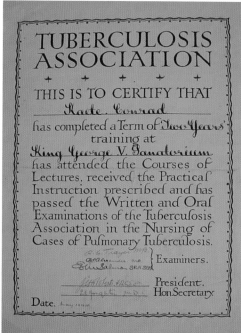

TUBERCULOSIS ASSOCIATION

+ + + + +

THIS IS TO CERTIFY THAT

Katie Conrad

has completed a Term of *Two Years'* training at

King George V. Sanatorium

has attended the Courses of Lectures, received the Practical Instruction prescribed and has passed the Written and Oral Examinations of the Tuberculosis Association in the Nursing of Cases of Pulmonary Tuberculosis.

} Examiners.

President.
Hon Secretary.

Date.

Above: Nurses manning a stand at a tuberculosis public health communication event in the West Midlands, *c.*1950s–60s. (Adrian Wressell, Heart of England NHS Foundation Trust)

Left: The British Tuberculosis Association was established in March 1928. The King George V Sanatorium, Hydestile, Surrey, where this nurse completed her training in 1944, had a reputation for being at the forefront of TB treatment and research, and was instrumental in pioneering development of drug therapy (streptomycin) to combat TB and the manufacture of iron lung equipment.

rest centre in an East London school, which was providing shelter for around 100 people who had been bombed out of their homes. When forty-five badly shocked people needed treating, there were cuts, scratches and lacerations to be dealt with, and days of caring for them as they recovered their equilibrium.

Tuberculosis spread like wildfire during the war years, due in part to poor living conditions, and, in the case of London, from people spending hours crowded into the underground Tube shelters. Staff Nurse Cissie Ridings encountered the disease for the first time in early 1945 at Ladywell Hospital, Eccles, near Salford. Patients from their teens to sixty spent anything from months to years there, and an abiding memory was of 'the dominant sound of coughing and spitting, followed by the clink of the sputum mug lids as they fell back in place. It was not a pleasant sound, but one I would grow accustomed to over this period'.

At the outbreak of war Queen Alexandra's Imperial Military Nursing Service (QAs) had around 624 members on active service in military hospitals, and they were called upon to nurse in battle areas around the world. They all had officer status, but were not commissioned until 1941, when emergency commissions were introduced and a rank structure established, which meant, for the first time, they could be promoted through the ranks up to brigadier, wear rank badges and be paid commensurately. As in the First World War, their numbers were boosted by the mobilisation of QA reservists and members of the Territorial Army Nursing Service (TANS), reaching a total of about 12,000 in 1945.

Did you know?

Nurses who joined the QAIMNS as reservists in 1938, in anticipation of war in Europe, were interviewed by the War Office and presented with a sealed envelope stating 'Open only in the event of war'.

Jessie Park Smith was a surgical ward sister when she signed up as a QA reservist in 1942, joining the 98th British General Hospital. From Algiers, then Chateaudun de Rumel (sic), she was sent, in December 1943, to Bari, southern Italy, and the so-called 3,000-bed Policlinic. The staff dealing with the mass of casualties affected by mustard gas burns had to wear gas masks and gloves, but the use of penicillin in treating these burns was a revelation. Jessie recounted, 'This was the first time that penicillin had been used on such a large scale and a real breakthrough in medicine.' And it was only due to the persuasive powers of the matron that she and her fellow sisters were allowed to administer the antibiotic hypodermically. Penicillin and sulphonamide were widely used in the Casualty Clearing Stations where Sister Eva Price served on the Western Front. She had been called up as a QA Reservist after the D-Day landings in June 1944, and remarked later that, 'When one is nursing the troops one can never fail to be impressed by their patience under wretched conditions, and that inextinguishable sense of humour that is always cropping up.' Yet another QA nurse, Sister Hannah Broadhead, survived the deliberate sinking of the hospital ship *Talamba*, on which she was serving in April 1943.

The navy and air force had their own nursing services whose numbers were boosted during the conflict by reservists and VADs. By the end of the war Princess Mary's Royal Air

Force Nursing Service's (est. 1918) numbers had increased from 171 to 1341, and Queen Alexandra's Royal Naval Nursing Service from seventy-eight members to 1,215.

Like the QAs, the naval nursing sisters experienced bombings and torpedoes, but also incarceration in a Japanese prison camp, and towards the end of the war played a part in the repatriation of patients from the Pacific Islands to Australia, America, Canada and India.

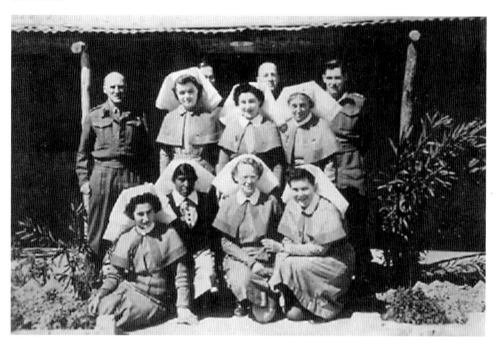

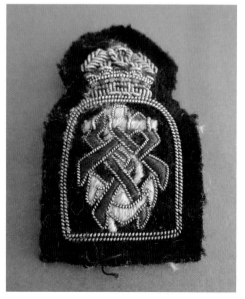

Above: Sister Kathleen Evans QAIMNS (R), kneeling second right in the front row, served in Palestine and Beirut during the Second World War. (Patricia Frearson)
Left: A Queen Alexandra's Royal Naval Nursing Service cap badge, n.d. (Peter Maleczek)

7
The NHS and Beyond

The end of the Second World War may have heralded a new era, but the country faced a shortage of nurses. To address this the Ministry of Health opened up the profession to male nurses, organising a special one-year course in general training for ex-servicemen who could meet stringent experience criteria. Those men who had less prior practice could enrol as assistant nurses. District nursing numbers were also down by around 500 in August 1947, so the introduction of training for male members of the QIDN was welcomed, and by 1958, 426 male SRNs had qualified as QNs. The introduction of the National Health Service in July 1948 changed the face of nursing care in the UK, exerting all kinds of new pressures on the profession. Every aspect of medical care and treatment was now free to everyone, regardless of

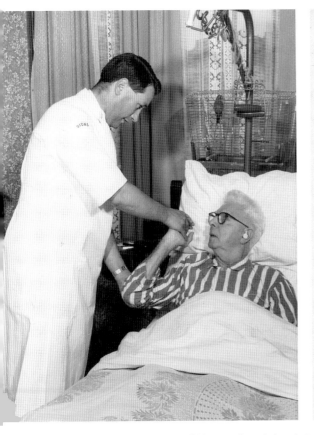

Nursing Mirror, February 3. 1950

GROWING IMPORTANCE of the MALE NURSE

Parliamentary Secretary, Ministry of Health, pays tribute at

SOCIETY OF REGISTERED MALE NURSES' A.G.M.

A LARGE gathering of male nurses from all parts of the country met at the Royal College of Nursing, London, last week for the Annual General Meeting of the Society of Registered Male Nurses. Mr. J. Sayer was re-elected as Chairman for the ensuing year, and Mr. F. A. W. Craddock was elected Secretary in the place of Mr. D. G. Melrose, who had resigned. Mr. G. Stainer's election as Treasurer which had taken place earlier in the year was confirmed, also that of Mr. J. H. Waitzer as Assistant Secretary. The following members were elected to the Executive Council: Messrs. D. G. Melrose, S. G. Bartlett, G. Wootton, W. G. Jones, W. Codd, D. T. Lewis, E. Dawson and W. Bushell. The vacancy created by Mr. Craddock's appointment was left until the Council met to decide who should serve on it. Mr. D. G. Melrose, Mr. F. A. W. Craddock, Mr. G. Stainer and Mr. J. H. Waitzer were thanked for their help during the past year.

In his report, Mr. Melrose, retiring secretary, said that " 1949 was another year of hard work on the part of the Executive Council of the Society. The Journal and monthly minutes have been circulated as usual to all members and student members. Once more thanks are due to the members of the Executive Council who assisted in the really large task of dispatching them. The Council is trying to do all possible to relieve the delay and improve the position during 1950."

Contact with various branches and units was made by a series of meetings at which Mr. Sayer spoke; these visits included Birmingham, Wolverhampton, Nuneaton, Nottingham and Leicester.

During the year Mr. Craddock resigned from the General Nursing Council, owing to the pressure of his personal duties. His place was taken by Mr. J. Sayer, the present Chairman of the Society. Mr. Dawson was appointed as a member of the Central Health Services Council.

Contacts and Representation

During the year Mr. Glavin, the founder member of the Society, emigrated to Australia. A presentation was made to him, in appreciation of his work for the Society. A letter has since been received from Mr. Glavin, describing his enthusiastic reception by the representatives of the male nurses of Western Australia when his ship called at Freemantle. Contact has been maintained throughout the

year with male nurses from Australia, New Zealand, South Africa, America, India and Malaya.

Not least of the activities of the Society has been the representation on the Nurses' Standing Committee of the Whitley Council. Some grades have received salary increases, and the Society's representative has played a part in obtaining these. The representative and the Executive Council are fully aware that anomalies exist, and are doing their best to remedy these. Satisfactory increases in other grades are hoped for in the near future.

The Society was asked to send representatives to the Canterbury Festival on the Science and Art of Healing. This was attended by several members and student members, including the Chairman and General Secretary. After the service the members were shown round the Cathedral.

The badges proposed at the last Annual General Meeting have now been prepared, and may be obtained from the Treasurer (*see illustrations at head of this page*).

After much consideration the Executive Council decided to withdraw affiliation with the National Council of Nurses, and this has since been done.

One of the most important events in the nursing world has been the passing of the Nurses Bill. The stages of this Bill have been closely watched by the Executive Council, and several recommendations were sent to the Minister. One of these was a protest against the deletion of the title of Chief Male Nurse; the representations of the Society were successful on this point, and the title has now been reinserted once more.

The Treasurer's report showed a balance of £215 9s. of income over expenditure.

Reorganisation of the Society

The Society of Registered Male Nurses is to be organised on a regional basis which is to come into force gradually through this year, and officially begin in January, 1951. The country will be divided into 10 regions for this purpose, as under the National Health Act. Each region will have a council consisting of members each representing 30 male nurses from the different branches. The council will have a chairman and secretary. Each region will nominate one member for a National Council which will deal only with

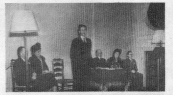

Parliamentary Secretary, Ministry of Health, Mr. Arthur Blenkinsop, M.P., addressing the Open Meeting of the Society's A.G.M. (left) and on the platform (left to right) Mr. G. Stainer, Miss Russell Smith, Mr. Blenkinsop, standing (hiding Mr. Sayer), Dr. Rees Thomas, Dame Louise Wilkinson, Mr. D. G. Melrose.

Above left: The new male QNs complained that their white coats had to be dry cleaned, but Raymond Philpot was more bothered by being regularly mistaken for the gasman, the meter reader and even a sailor. (QNI)

Above right: An article on the importance of male nurses. *Nursing Mirror*, 3 February 1950.

their financial circumstances, creating a greater demand for qualified nurses, who were already in short supply. Even though the training for the lower grade of state-enrolled assistant nurse, introduced in 1948, was shorter than for registered nurses, it failed to attract enough recruits.

There were also increasing concerns over the standard of training and low level of education amongst trainees, which was blamed on the Ministry of Health's decision in 1939 to suspend the General Nursing Council's minimum standards. Whilst the major teaching hospitals set their own entry standard criteria, smaller hospitals were less fussy and took on students who struggled to pass the GNC exam. These factors led the two most senior sister tutors in the country to argue, in 1951, that:

> Shortages will never be overcome by reducing the standard of candidates to the nursing profession, or by exploiting during training those who have come forward ... [it it] only a matter of time before we regress to the standard of Sairey Gamp and Betsy Prig.

Yet another problem was the lack of well-trained tutors. The GNC hoped by introducing a requirement, after 1946, that only nurses who had completed their prescribed course (available at six universities around England) could be registered as tutors, and would raise standards. However, as hospitals were under no obligation to employ qualified tutors, the take-up was low. Up until 1959 the only choice for those in England who wanted a route into nurse teaching was the postal Diploma in Nursing course, run by the University of London since 1925. It did attract more academic women, including Margaret Lamb, who compared it to the Open University, and thoroughly enjoyed the challenge.

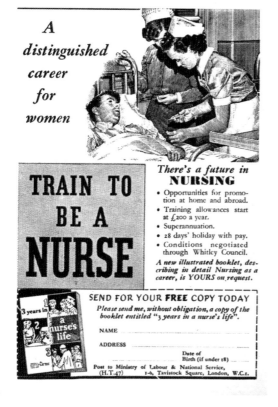

Student nurses were less than happy with one aspect of the new NHS for when they received their wage packets from their new employer in July 1948 they were dismayed to find themselves worse off than before. Living on a student nurses' salary of £3 3s 4d a month was hard enough, but to find that they had 10s a month deducted for National Insurance and superannuation contributions was just too much to bear, and led to a public protest march in London in the August and a threatened strike. By the end of 1948 nurses' pay was increased by £8 a month, and the numbers belonging to the

This 'Train to be a Nurse' poster was published by the Ministry of Labour in 1952. (Yahoo Flickr)

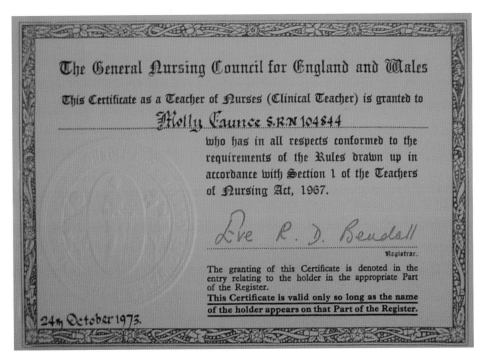

GNC certificate for a teacher of nurses, 1973.

GNC certificate for a nurse tutor, 1959.

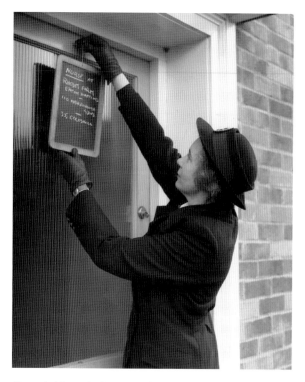

Queen's Nurse Jeal writing the details of the patients she was visiting on a slate outside her home. This way she could be reached in the case of an emergency. (QNI)

Student Nurses' Association rose sharply to 19,000. The burning question of equal pay for male and female nurses raged for years until 1955, when the Conservative government agreed to introduce public service equal pay, phased in over six years.

Nurses certainly welcomed the end of fundraising and encouraging donations and subscriptions, which had been essential pre-NHS to maintain voluntary hospitals and district nursing associations. District nurses were especially pleased, for many, including Irene Sankey, had found asking for money 'embarrassing and distasteful, asking them about their income and expenditure'. Another step forward was that every district case could now have a nurse and a doctor if need be. Communication, which was vital for the district nurse, became easier as the 1950s rolled in. Public telephone kiosks became more commonplace and telephones were installed in private houses and district nurses' homes, and in the late 1960s the introduction of the car radio telephone meant that instant communication was possible.

Did you know?

In April 1950, Eric and Edith Willis got married and became the first NHS nurses to be allowed to live together outside the standard nurses' quarters. The pair had met during their training at the Preliminary Training School of Derbyshire Royal Infirmary in 1948 – the year the NHS was founded. They started dating a year later and when they fell in love, their matron gave permission for them to break with tradition and live outside the hospital grounds once they were married.

Post-NHS, the College of Nursing stuck to their traditional view that three or four years' apprenticeship was the ideal period for SRNs, and in 1959, when Marion Kirby trained, little had changed. She started as a trainee nurse with seven others in Chertsey, Surrey, and spent her first twelve weeks of training at Highfield House in West Byfleet, where the girls shared rooms.

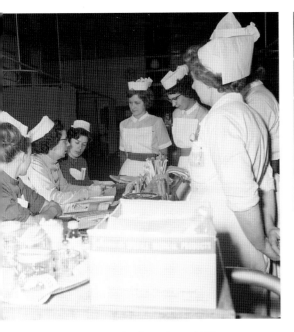

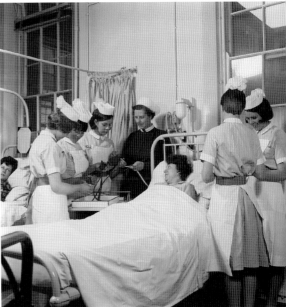

Above left: Staff handover, 1950s.
Above right: Nurses receiving bedside teaching, c.1950s. (Peter Maleczek)

The 'domestic' tasks after breakfast were still there, from sweeping floors to cleaning bathrooms and bed making, ready for matron's inspection and the doctor's round. After that:

> We'd go off to class for anatomy, physiology or practical skills lessons. Practical skills took place inside a 'mock' ward and we'd learn how to roll bandages and make beds hospital envelope corners. Our patient was a female dummy. We practised taking each other's blood pressure and used to lift and turn one another as we would the patients. Injections were performed on an orange. We'd spend one day every week on the wards at St. Peter's Hospital in Surrey.

The highlight for Zena Edmund-Jones, who came to England from Jamaica in 1956 to train as a nurse, were 'the day trips to places such as Oxo, Glaxo and the sewage works. I loved the day out, the teas, the little gifts – but not parts of the sewage works!' She also recalled her work and wage pattern: 'Forty-four hours per week were worked. I had one day off weekly and two weeks' holiday per year. Each nurse spent three months in each of the three years training on night duty. Wages were £10 per month for first year staff in the 1950s.'

As the 1960s dawned, change was on the way. The membership of the RCN stood at 43,000 but within twelve years had reached nearly 90,000. New minimum entry requirements were introduced that addressed earlier concerns over entry standards, so that prospective SRNs had to have five O levels, and the renamed state-enrolled nurse (SEN) needed at least two O levels. By the 1970s more and more SENs were working within the NHS, often undertaking the same type of work as a staff nurse, but without the recognition or career prospects. New courses became available, including the combined SRN/Registered

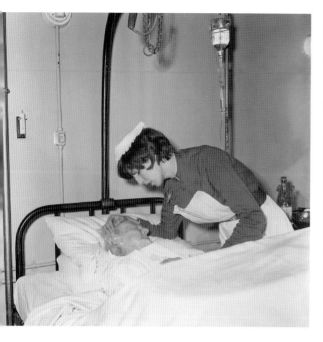

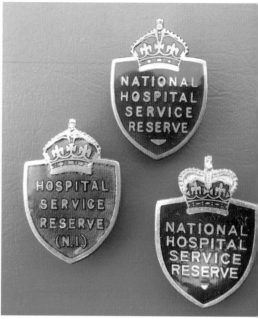

ALL REPLIES TO
MISS A. M. JOHNSON
MATRON

TELEPHONE Nº
HOP 7600

MATRON'S OFFICE

GUY'S HOSPITAL
LONDON
S·E·1

Ref.: JMH

26th October, 1964.

Miss S. Bennett,
Derlwyn Home Farm,
Alihoalis,
CARMARTHEN, S. Wales.

Dear   Miss Bennett,

In reply to your letter, I have pleasure in enclosing a prospectus of the Guy's Hospital School of Nursing, together with the necessary application papers. Would you please complete and return these to me as soon as possible, together with:

(a) Your Birth Certificate.

(b) A signed statement from your Headmistress in respect of the subjects which you have passed for the General Certificate of Education.

(c) An essay on "A Hobby", "A Holiday" or "Occupation since leaving School".

I will be glad to consider your application further, and, if this is satisfactory, to arrange for a personal interview. Final acceptance is always subject to a satisfactory medical examination held at Guy's within six months of entry.

Yours sincerely,

Administrative Sister.
pp.   Matron.

M.O.7.

Left: The National Hospital Service Reserve operated between 1949 and 1968, and was established in response to the Cold War and the threat of nuclear proliferation. The staff were uniformed volunteers from the nursing and medical professions, most of whom were either registered or auxiliary nurses.
Above right: National Hospital Service Reserve badges.
Above left: A nurse and elderly patient, 1950s.
(Peter Maleczek)

Mental Nurse qualification, and as new medical procedures were introduced, sophisticated nursing skills were required. When the London Hospital opened its first intensive care unit in 1965, nurses were thrown in at the deep end, and Carol recalled encountering her first ever ventilator and being terrified that something would happen to the patient.

Did you know?

Advance nurse practitioners are experienced and highly educated SRNs who oversee the complete clinical care of patients. They are able to assess, investigate, diagnose and prescribe medication.

The greatest change to nurse education came in 1993, when Project 2000 became fully operational. The new system phased out the enrolled nurse qualification and did away with the old apprenticeship model, with training moved out of schools attached to hospitals and into universities. Instead of learning as they worked, studying was moved elsewhere, with a diploma or a degree at the end. In 2009, the then Health Minister, Ann Keen, announced that from 2013 nursing was to become an all-graduate profession, prompting a variety of responses for and against the change. One student nurse, Sarah, could not see a problem, saying, 'If people are serious and dedicated to becoming a nurse I do not see why this would discourage them from entering the profession. Whether you are "academic" or not, you still have assignments and exams when you enter nursing education.'

In 2019 the RCN could claim to be 'the world's largest nursing union and professional body, representing over 400,000 registered nurses, midwives and health care assistants in the UK and internationally, as well as around 35,000 nursing students'. There is now a new generation of nurses caring for sick people in the community, whose profile as professionals has been raised beyond recognition since the days of Florence Nightingale and her contemporary nursing reform pioneers. What has not changed is the need and desire to provide their patients with the best possible care.

A female nurse carries out observations on a male inpatient. The patient is in bed in a UK hospital ward. The nurse is measuring the patient's blood-oxygen levels. The nurse is a staff nurse and wears a pale blue uniform with white trim. (Adrian Wressell, Heart of England NHS Foundation Trust)

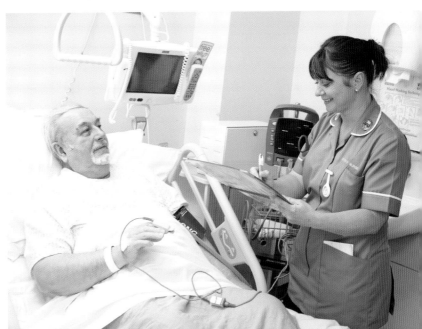

8

What Now?

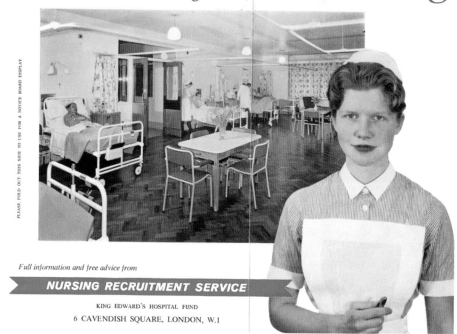

Your Life in Nursing

PLEASE FOLD OUT THIS SIDE TO USE FOR A NOTICE BOARD DISPLAY

Full information and free advice from

NURSING RECRUITMENT SERVICE

KING EDWARD'S HOSPITAL FUND
6 CAVENDISH SQUARE, LONDON, W.1

Advertising leaflet, *c*.1950s/60s. (Peter Maleczek)

Researching Nurses and Nursing History

Whether you are a genealogist or just interested in knowing more about the nursing profession, there is a wealth of resources available to help you find out about individual nurses, the organisations they belonged to, and the places where they worked.

Oral history has come to play a very large part in retelling the story of individual nurses and their experiences, and there are many recordings available for you to listen to and text for you to read.

The Kingston and St George's nursing oral history project 'Nurses Voices' has memories of nurses working on the wards in the 1940s and 1950s at St George's at Christmastime and during the Second World War. These can be heard on YouTube at www.youtube.com/watch?v=S-CrycmFa4U&feature=youtu.be.

The British Library Sound and Moving Image Archive has numerous collections of interviews, which can be listened to at the British Library Reading Rooms in London and

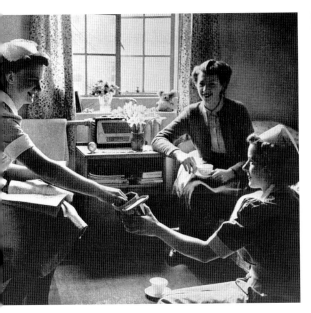
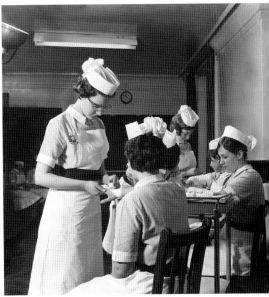

***Above left**: Off-duty nurses in Birmingham, c.1950s–60s. (Rob McRorie)*
***Above right**: Nurses practising their bandaging skills, c.1950s–60s. (Peter Maleczek)*

Yorkshire. You will need to search the Sound and Moving Image catalogue to find the recording you want, make a note of the shelfmark, and contact the library with the details. You will find the shelfmark at the top of each entry in the catalogue.

To book an appointment telephone 020 7412 7418, email Listening@bl.uk or visit www.bl.uk/help/listening-and-viewing-service.

These include Andy Stevens' psychiatric nursing interviews, recorded circa 1991; focus on former nursing employees working at Essex Hall/Turner village in Essex; and the Hallam Nursing Interviews, recorded in 1992 to 1993, the memories of four women who came from Barbados to train as nurses in Britain in the 1950s. The Royal College of Nursing History Group has recordings of thirty-five interviews with nurses.

The Royal College of Nursing Oral History Collection has over 600 recordings of individuals trained between 1910 and the 1950s. Most of the collection is available as a digital recording and transcript, and can accessed either at the Royal College of Nursing Archives, No. 42 South Oswald Road, Edinburgh, EH9 2HH. Tel: 0345 337 3368. www.rcn.org.uk/library/archives. E-mail archives@rcn.org.uk. Opening hours are Monday to Friday 9.00 a.m. to 5.00 p.m. Closed 25 December to 3 January. Advance booking and proof of identity required.

Or at the Royal College of Nursing and Heritage Centre, No. 20 Cavendish Square, London, W1G 0RN. Tel: 034 533 73368. Email rcn.library@rcn.org.uk.

The Memories of Nursing Project captured 'stories of the professional lives of a group of ageing nurses', many of whom were working before and during the Second World War, and recalled the early days of the NHS. memoriesofnursing.uk/nursing-archive.

Imperial War Museum on-line collections includes many oral nursing histories: www.iwm.org.uk.

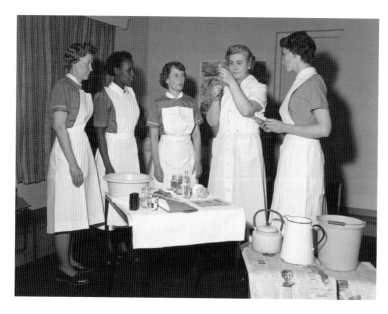

Nurses being trained to use a hypodermic syringe, 1960s.

Historic nursing journals are a rich source of information on individual nurses, as well as the organisations and their workings. Several libraries have runs of historic nursing magazines, which can be viewed once you have obtained a reader's ticket.

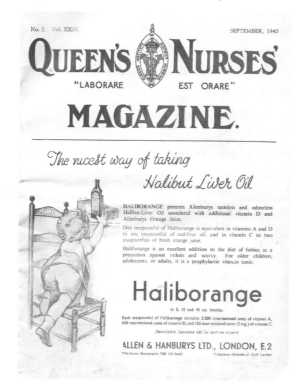

Left and opposite: Nursing magazines.

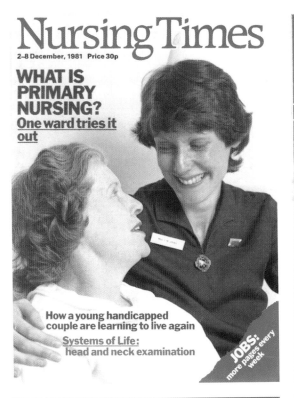

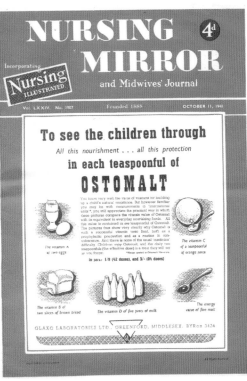

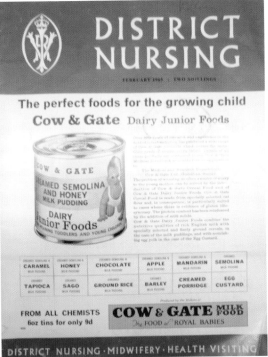

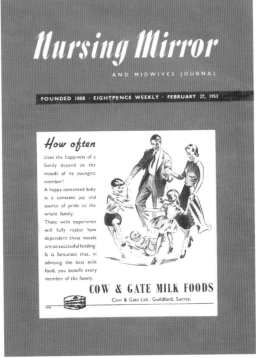

Nursing Journals

The British Library Reading Rooms, No. 96 Euston Road, London, NW1 2DB
Tel: Customer Services: +44 (0)1937 546060. Email: Customer-Services@bl.uk. Opening hours: Monday 10.00 a.m. to 8:00 p.m., Tuesday to Thursday 9.30 a.m. to 8.00 p.m., Friday & Saturday 9.30 a.m. to 5.00 p.m. www.bl.uk.

Wellcome Library, Wellcome Collection, No. 183 Euston Road, London, NW1 2BE. Tel: 020 7611 8722. Email: library@wellcome.ac.uk. Opening hours: Monday, Tuesday, Wednesday, Friday 10.00 a.m. to 6.00 p.m., Thursday 10.00 a.m. to 8.00 p.m., Saturday 10.00 a.m. to 4.00 p.m. Closed Sundays and all bank holidays. www.wellcomelibrary.org.

The Royal College of Nursing has a complete digitised run of the *Nursing Record/British Journal of Nursing* from 1888–1956 available to research on-line: rcnarchive.rcn.org.

Places to Visit to Research Nurses and Nursing

The National Archives, Kew, Richmond, TW9 4DU. Tel: 020 8876 3444. Opening hours: Tuesday to Saturday 9.30 a.m. to 4.00 p.m. Closed Sunday and Monday and bank holidays. A reader's ticket is needed and you can pre-register for this on-line at https://secure.nationalarchives.gov.uk/login/yourdetails. There is a restaurant and café on site. www.nationalarchives.gov.uk.

The NA is a rich source of information about civilian, district and wartime nursing. Here you can find the records of the General Nursing Council for England and Wales, which includes the Register of Nurses 1921–73, the Roll of Nurses 1944–73 and the computerised register and roll for 1973–83. The register will provide details of the date and place of qualification for every nurse. If you know which hospital a nurse worked in, then the Hospital Records Database should be your first port of call. You'll be able to find out whether any records have survived for the hospital, and where these are located. The database can be found at www.nationalarchives.gov.uk/hospitalrecords.

The NA also hold 15,000 service records for the First World War period. These records could reveal where a nurse trained pre-war, how suitable she was considered to be for military service, where she served and when she left the service. There may also be a superintendent's report, which would have been confidential: www.nationalarchives.gov.uk/help-with-your-research/research-guides/british-army-nurses-service-records-1914-1918.

A search of the NA catalogue will provide you with details of numerous records held on site relating to local district nursing associations, including some belonging to the Queen's Nursing Institute, as well as information about similar material held in local archives across the UK.

London Metropolitan Archives, No. 40 Northampton Road, Clerkenwell, London, EC1R 0HB. Tel: 020 7332 3820. Email: asklma@cityoflondon.gov.uk. For Information Leaflet No. 36 History of Nursing: www.cityoflondon.gov.uk/things-to-do/london-metropolitan-archives/visitor-information/Documents/36-history-of-nursing-at-lma.pdf.

Amongst the archive collection are Florence Nightingale's papers and those of the Nightingale School and Nightingale Fund Council. Register for a History Card online, to access archive material. Opening times are 9.30 a.m. to 4.45 p.m. Monday to Thursday, with a late closing on Wednesday at 7.30 p.m. Check the website for once-a-month Saturday opening dates. Closed all bank holidays.

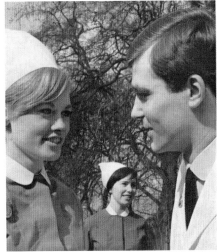

A career for men and women

PSYCHIATRIC NURSING

of mentally ill or
mentally subnormal people

"Nursing — surely the most
rewarding job in the world"

Training poster for
psychiatric nurses,
c.1960s–70s.

An entry from the Queen's Roll for Grace Hardy, appointed Queen's Nurse in 1905. She trained for four years as a nurse in Dublin before undertaking her six months of district training. Inspectors always complimented her on being 'kind, tactful and sympathetic', but from 1919 remarked that her actual nursing methods were 'out of date'. She was awarded her long-service medal in 1926. (Wellcome Library, London)

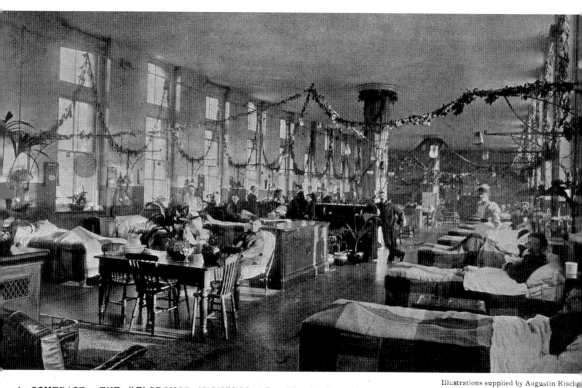

Illustrations supplied by Augustin Rischg

A CONTRAST: THE "FLORENCE NIGHTINGALE" WARD IN ST. THOMAS'S HOSPITAL, WESTMINSTER
Miss Florence Nightingale, who was born at Florence on May 12th, 1820, is a Lady of Grace of St. John of Jerusalem

Florence Nightingale Ward, St Thomas's Hospital, London, c. Christmas 1914.

The Queen's Nursing Institute Archive (SA/QNI) can be found at the Wellcome Library, Special Collections, Rare Materials Reading Room, No. 183 Euston Road, London, NW1 2BE. Tel: 020 7611 8722. Email: collections@wellcome.ac.uk. Opening hours: Monday, Tuesday, Wednesday, Friday 10.00 a.m. to 6.00 p.m., Thursday 10.00 a.m. to 8.00 p.m., Saturday 10.00 a.m. to 4.00 p.m. Closed Sundays and all bank holidays. This is an extensive and comprehensive archive that covers every aspect of the organisation, including the Roll of Nurses. You can, for example, search for a Queen's Nurse by name or roll number and trace a nurse's history from a badge number. archives.wellcomelibrary.org.

Places to Visit

Florence Nightingale Museum, St Thomas' Hospital, No. 21 Lambeth Palace Road, London, SE1 7EW. Tel: 020 7188 4400. www.florence-nightingale.co.uk.

The museum celebrates the life and work of Miss Nightingale and has a huge collection of personal items, letters, nursing memorabilia and Crimean War artefacts. Entry charge applies. Guided tours and group visits can be arranged. Opening times: Daily 10.00 a.m. to 5.00 p.m. (last entry 4.30 p.m. Check the website for bank holiday closures and admission charge.

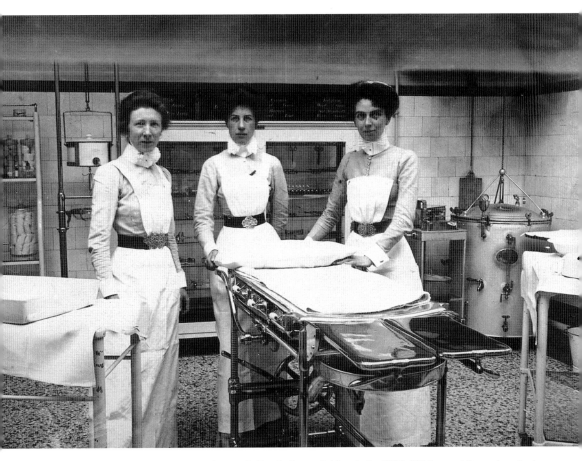

London nurses in the operating theatre, St Bartholomew's Hospital, *c.*1905. (Wellcome Library, London)

British Red Cross Museum and Archives, No. 44 Moorfields, London, EC2Y 9AL. Tours and research appointments which must be made in advance by emailing enquiry@ redcross.org.uk, are available 10.00 a.m. to 4.00 p.m. Monday to Thursday.

A total of 90,000 people were volunteers with the BRC during the First World War, and you can search the on-line catalogue by individual name or that of a Red Cross Hospital. www.redcross.org.uk/WW1.

Royal College of Nursing and Heritage Centre. No. 20 Cavendish Square, London, W1G 0RN. Tel: 034 533 73368. Email rcn.library@rcn.org.uk. There are regularly changing exhibitions on display in the heritage centre, and the RCN holds regular events.

The Royal London Hospital Museum and Archives, St Augustine with St Phillip's Church, Newark Street, London, E1 2AA. Tel: 020 7377 7608. The archive and museum collections include material relating to key figures in nursing history including Edith Cavell and hospital matron Eva Luckes. Open Tuesday to Friday, from 10 a.m.–4 p.m. Closed over Christmas, New Year, Easter and public holidays.

St Bartholomew's Hospital Museum and Archives, North Wing, West Smithfield, London, EC1A 7BE. Tel: 020 3465 5798. E-mail: barts.archives@bartshealth.nhs.uk. www.bartshealth.nhs.uk/the-royal-london-hospital-museum-and-archives

The museum charts nine centuries of healthcare, and the collections and objects highlight the changes in the care of patients and the training of staff.

Open Tuesday to Friday, from 10.00 a.m.–4.00 p.m. Closed over Christmas, New Year, Easter and public holidays.

The Museum of Military Medicine, Keogh Barracks, Ash Vale, Aldershot, GU12 5RQ. Tel: 01252 868612. Open daily Monday to Friday 9.30 a.m. to 3.30 p.m. Closed bank holidays. Free admission.

Websites
The Queen's Nursing Institute's heritage website is a unique interactive resource where you can explore stories and memories of district nurses, and view films and photos from their archive. The QNI do not hold any archive material. https://qniheritage.org.uk.

Scarlet Finders is an excellent resource for researching nurses connected to the military nursing services. www.scarletfinders.co.uk.

Further Reading
Whether you are interested in the history of nursing for specific reasons or out of general interest, the range of reading material available is legion. Some of these are listed here:

Boase, Anne, Bellman, Loretta, Rodgers, Sarah and Stuchfield, Barbara, *Nursing Through the Years. Care and Compassion at the Royal London Hospital* (Yorkshire, Pen & Sword History, 2019). A unique history of eighty years of the Royal London Hospital through memories of the nurses who worked there.

Ardern, Peter, *When Matron Ruled* (London, Robert Hale, 2002). Includes many direct accounts from matrons, who were both loved and feared.

Baly, Monica E., *A History of the Queen's Nursing Institute: 100 years 1887–1987* (London, Croom Helm, 1987). Traces the history of nursing the sick poor in their homes, showing what district nurses actually did.

McGann, Susan, Crowther, Anne and Dougall, Rona, *A History of the Royal College of Nursing 1916–90: A Voice for Nurses* (Manchester, Manchester University Press, 2009). A history of professional nursing from 1916, drawn from the archives of the Royal College of Nursing.

Piggott, Juliet, *Queen Alexandra's Royal Army Nursing Corps* (London, Leo Cooper Ltd, 1975) An account of the development of the military nursing service.

Powell, Anne, *Women in the War Zone: Hospital Services in the First World* War (Stroud, Gloucs. The History Press, 2009). A rich selection of personal accounts of First World War nurses.